T0320889

LOSING TOUCH

JONATHAN COLE

LOSING TOUCH

A Man Without his Body

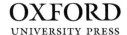

OXFORD
UNIVERSITY PRESS

Great Clarendon Street, Oxford, OX2 6DP,
United Kingdom

Oxford University Press is a department of the University of Oxford.
It furthers the University's objective of excellence in research, scholarship,
and education by publishing worldwide. Oxford is a registered trade mark of
Oxford University Press in the UK and in certain other countries

First Edition published in 2016
Impression: 1

Published in the United States of America by Oxford University Press
198 Madison Avenue, New York, NY 10016, United States of America

British Library Cataloguing in Publication Data
Data available

Library of Congress Control Number: 2016942681

ISBN 978–0–19–877887–5

Printed and bound by
CPI Group (UK) Ltd, Croydon, CR0 4YY

To colleagues, for their curiosity and friendship

ACKNOWLEDGEMENTS

This book is about how we can understand living with the loss of cutaneous touch and movement/position sense or proprioception, which happened to Ian Waterman when he was 19, 45 years ago now. The answers come both from scientific experiment and from a more personal, first-person biographical exploration of how Ian has managed.

The book covers around 30 years of research with Ian, and throughout that period he has consented to experiments, involving varying degrees of intrusion, boredom, pain, and pleasure, with enthusiasm and curiosity. More than that, he has become an expert in neuroscience himself, often knowing as much or more than the scientists he meets about how to design a good experiment. He has also put up with decades of questions from intrigued scientists about how he does so and so and what he feels about that, with grace and humor.

In parallel with our scientific experiments, he has also been prepared to explore and make available his personal experiences and reflections about living for so long without the sensations from his body that almost everyone else takes for granted. Only by his own, first-person, reflections do we gain another level of understanding. And this has come from conversations over many years between us, at our homes and on the road as we ourselves went from being young men, through middle age, to being grandparents. In addition to these we have also sat in more directed sessions at Ian's home going through his life and views on science and scientists over many days and weeks during the last few years.

So, my first and most important acknowledgment and thanks go to Ian for engaging with science, and for allowing his biographical details to be mingled with his reflections on living without touch and proprioception. Thanks also for his company over many years and for trusting me with both the science and with his biography.

I occasionally act as a medical opinion for Ian; he is the subject of experiments I develop or arrange and am involved in, I have become his biographer and am his friend. It is my hope that we have managed to separate these, and that my present role is as an independent observer and chronicler, off-camera, audio-recorder to hand. We are both quite clear that the science has to be done objectively, though that objectivity includes Ian's observations of his methods and bodily response. When considering his first-person experiences, and how much personal detail he wants to divulge, the line might be difficult to draw since the illness has reached into many parts of his life. But he has controlled the content throughout.

Much of the biographical material in this book was discussed at Ian's house in Dorset, assisted by his wife, Brenda. It is a pleasure to thank her for her support, for acting as Ian's PA during research trips, and for her constant supply of tea, cakes, lunches, and common sense.

Research papers reflect ideas and hunches and reveal results, concepts, and predictions; what is not apparent is that science is a human endeavor, and like all endeavors there are periods of frustration, of boredom, as well as of elation. People do research because they are intrigued and curious, a wonderful mind set both to be in and to see in others. It has therefore been a privilege, and hugely enjoyable, to have been involved in, and stimulated by, research with Ian in a number of labs over the years. A visit to a lab is not just about science, we have received kindness and consideration everywhere we have been and enjoyed times in the bar after experiments and day excursions fitted in round experiments to fascinating places. Thanks are due to a huge number of clinicians and scientists, philosophers and psychologists, as well as those in theater, television, and choreography.

Our first research in Southampton was with Haider Katifi, Malcolm Burnett, Mike Sedgwick, and Louis Merton. At Laval in Quebec the team who had done months of planning to make the visits such a success included Chantal Bard, Michelle Fleury, Yves Lamarre, Normand Teasdale, Jean Blouin, Yves Lajoie, and Jacques Paillard, while in Marseille we worked with Gabriel Gauthier, Jean-Louis Vercher, Olivier Guedon, and Magali Billon. More recently we have also collaborated there with Fabrice Sarlegna, Hannah Lefumat, Frank Buloup, Lionel Bringoux, and Christophe Bourdin, and with Gavin Buckingham then in Edinburgh. In Seeweisen, Germany, thanks are due to Horst Mittelstaedt and in Hamburg (then) Rolf-Detlef Treede.

From University College London thanks are due to Patrick Haggard, John Rothwell, and Brian Day for several projects over many years and to Flavia Mancini, Gian Domenico Iannetti, Nada Yousif, Joern Diedrichsen, Richard Fitzpatrick, and Billy Luu. Another long-term collaborator has been Chris Miall in Birmingham with mention also to Daniela Balslev.

Investigation of affective touch centered on Goteborg thanks to Håkan Olausson and Francis McGlone (from Liverpool John Moores University), together with Åke Vallbo, Catherine Bushnell, Mikael Elam, and Jaquette Liljencrantz. Further work followed in Helsinki with Gina Caetano and Riita Hari. Work on affective proprioception was written with Barbara Montero from New York.

In the early 1990s I was invited by Tony Marcel to a week-long seminar on neuroscience and philosophy in King's College, Cambridge, and there I met a phenomenologist, Shaun Gallagher. Through him I have also met others interested in what might be called the first-person approach, including Dan Zahavi in Copenhagen. I thank both for many fruitful discussions over the years. It was through Shaun that our research on gesture with David McNeill was initiated, and through David we also worked with Liesbet Quaeghebeur and Susan Duncan.

We made several visits to the Max Planck Institute, which was then in Munich. It is a pleasure to thank Simone Bosbach-Schulz, Wolfgang Prinz, Günther Knoblich, Prisca Stenneken, and Gisa Aschersleben. Similarly thanks to Joachim Hermsdörfer, Dennis Nowak, and their team from Munich, Arjan ter Horst, Rob van Lier, and Bert Steenbergen from Nijmegen, the Netherlands, Richard af Klint, Jens Bo Nielsen, Thomas Sinkjær, and Michael Grey in Aalborg, Denmark and, in Lyon, Pierre Fourneret and Marc Jeannerod. The absence of many of these names and the work done with them from *Losing Touch* does not reflect the quality of their science with Ian. It was simply that these visits did not illuminate Ian's scientific biographical development the way other trips did. Inevitably some work has not made it to finished papers, despite its importance. Thanks are due to Jim Lackner and Paul DiZio at Brandeis University in Boston for their work in relation to microgravity, to the late Abe Guz, together with Kevin Murphy, at Imperial College London, for work on the perception of breathing, and to Bal Athwal, Daniel Wolpert, Christopher Frith, and Richard Frakowiak, all then at University College London, for PET studies.

The shoots to make the BBC *Horizon* documentary were made by the team of Chris Rawlence, Emma Crichton-Miller, Sophie Weitzman, Chris Morphet, and Trevor Hotz. At times uncovering Ian's early period with the illness was difficult, but their good humor and support made it rewarding for Ian as well as—it is hoped—for viewers. Parts of the filming were facilitated by Marsha Ivins, (ex-NASA) and it is a pleasure to thank her for her support and encouragement. Ian's two portrayals in theater, parts of *L'Homme Qui* and *The Valley of Astonishment* were by David Bennent, Bruce Myers, and Marcello Magni. Thanks, above all, though for these to Peter Brook and Marie-Hélène Estienne. I am also grateful to Bloomsbury Methuen Drama for permission to quote from *The Man Who*. In choreography we have had the pleasure of working with Siobhan Davies and Matthias Sperling. Both these projects overlapped with work with Oliver Sacks. He was a mentor and friend for longer than I have known Ian, since I studied with him as a medical student in the mid-1970s, and his death in August 2015 robbed us of his unique curiosity, eloquence, and humanity.

ACKNOWLEDGEMENTS

In the Afterword several colleagues from the sciences and humanities write on their perceptions on working with Ian, leaving aside their usual professional objectivity for a short time. I am very grateful to them all for doing this so readily and thank Peter Brook, Emma Crichton-Miller, Siobhan Davies, Brian Day, Shaun Gallagher, Patrick Haggard, Francis McGlone, David McNeill, Chris Miall, Mark Mitton, and Håkan Olausson.

One consequence of Ian's neuronopathy becoming more widely known is that we have met several people with similar conditions, sometimes in scientific contexts but sometimes also for mutual support and advice. Thanks are due to Charles Freed, Ginette Lizotte (who like Ian has contributed hugely with her time and effort in research), and Jacqueline McCoy.

Huge thanks are due to Martin Baum at OUP for agreeing to publish the work (and for finding reviewers sympathetic to such a biographical scientific approach), to Catherine Dalzell and Sanjana Sundaram for their work on production, and to Bridget Johnson for her skill in editing. They made the work never less than a pleasure.

Most of the photographs are mine, but thanks to Chris Rawlence for permission to use one of us larking around in New York (a long time ago now) and to my wife for taking the photo of Ian and me at his wedding.

Lastly my thanks are due to my wife Sue and our daughters (in alphabetical order) Celia, Eleanor, Georgia, and Lydia for their support during the long process of writing, which was usually in the evenings and weekends. Though Sue is used to it by now and our girls grown up, their continuing encouragement is richly appreciated.

Jonathan Cole
Minstead, Hampshire
December 2015

CONTENTS

LIST OF ILLUSTRATIONS AND FIGURES

Illustrations

1. Ian during experiments. (a) On the catwalk in Laval University, Quebec, to investigate his attention towards walking. (b) In the circulating chamber at Brandeis University, Boston, for experiments on reaching during Coriolis forces, 1998. (c) Ian at the table for the turn and point experiment, Brandeis University, Boston, 1998. (d) Ian and Jonathan in KC135, the "Vomit Comet," Houston, 1998 (NASA). (e) Gait study, Aalborg, Denmark, 2007. (f) Magnetoencephalography, Helsinki, Finland, 2009. (g) Study of grasping, Birmingham, UK, 2012. (h) Study on reaching, University College London, 2013.
2. NASA DART robot. Once you were rigged in the gloves and with sensors on your arms, the robot moved as you moved and you saw the robot's arms in the head-mounted display via cameras in the robot's eyes, 1997.
3. The romance of filming. (a) Ian and Felice standing on a busy road in Jersey, in the rain, looking across at his old hospital ward, 1997. (b) Ian resting in between filming in the grounds of Salisbury Hospital. Chris Rawlence, the director, is taking the still photo and Chris Morphet, the cameraman, is measuring the light before starting filming. Ian was tired, but still playing to the camera, 1997. (c) Ian and Jonathan while filming in New York, 1997.
4. Ian and Oliver Sacks, in Florida, 1997.
5. Ian and Herb Schaumburg, New York City, 1997.
6. Ian and Brenda at their wedding, 2013.
7. Ian at the Museum of Modern Art, New York, 2013.
8. Ian instructing Matthias Sperling how to stand up for Siobhan Davies' and Matthias' *Manual*, 2014 (composite).
9. Ian during a Kohnstamm experiment in his kitchen, 2013.

Figure

Defects, disorders, diseases . . . can play a paradoxical role, by bringing out latent powers, development, evolutions, forms of life, that might never be seen, or even imaginable, in their absence . . . the paradox of disease [is] its "creative" potential.

The study of disease, for the physician, demands the study of identity, the inner worlds that patients, under the spur of illness, create. But . . . these worlds cannot be comprehended wholly from the observation of behaviour, from the outside. In addition to the objective approach of the scientist, we must employ an intersubjective approach, to see the world with the eyes of the patient himself.

—Oliver Sacks

Familiarity with the natural sciences and with scientific method has always kept me on my guard, and I have always tried where it was possible to be consistent with the facts of science, and where it was impossible I have preferred not to write at all.

—Anton Chekhov

INTRODUCTION

In 1971, aged 19, Ian Waterman contracted a gastric upset, an illness which changed the course of his life and has influenced the neuroscience of movement.

He had just left home to work as an apprentice butcher in Jersey, a British Channel Island, and was living in lodgings when he developed diarrhea. After a couple of days he was too weak to carry on. A friend's GP gave him a prescription, but at the chemist's he was so ill he needed help back into the car. He remembers little of the next few days. A doctor was sent for, arrived in his Bentley, shouted something from the car, and drove off. A day or so later his landlady offered to change his sheets. As Ian got out of bed he fell in a heap by a radiator. The landlady phoned for another doctor, who examined Ian and immediately admitted him to hospital.

By then his speech was slurred, he had a buzzing feeling in his hands, feet, and round his neck, and from his neck down he could feel nothing. He was asked to change into pajamas; the nurse returned to find he had not moved and scolded him. But he could no longer *do* anything; he just could not make his limbs do what he wanted. A doctor arrived and, focusing on Ian's slurred speech, assumed he was drunk. He examined Ian and realized it was more than alcohol, even though he had no idea what it was.

That evening Ian began to take stock. His whole body from the neck down was numb and he could not feel his tongue and the bottom of his mouth. Weird though this was, what was even odder was that he had no idea where his arms and legs were without looking. He was not paralyzed; his limbs moved, but he had no control over how and where they moved. That was why he had fallen so badly getting out of bed and why the radiator had felt warm rather than hard—he could no longer feel "hard" at all. Numb from the neck down, and with the back of his head numb too, he lay there feeling as though he was floating on the sheets he could not feel. At that point, unable to feel or move, he felt completely disembodied, he had lost touch—literally—with his own body; if he did not look, he did not know it was there. He was without his body in the sense that he could no longer make use of it, as a singer cannot sing without their voice. He was also terrified.

Next day the consultant came, but was non-committal. They wondered about Guillain–Barré syndrome, a form of acute post-infectious nerve disease, but the tests came back negative. It turned out that Ian's white blood cells had produced an antibody against the virus causing the diarrhea, which had reacted, in turn, with his nerve cells in a very specific, severe, and astonishingly rare way. In those few days it had destroyed—permanently—the sensory nerves underpinning touch and the sense of movement and position (or proprioception), from a level around the neck, leaving intact those nerves underpinning the sensations of temperature and pain and the motor nerves involved in movement. The damage was to the nerve cell bodies in the small dorsal root ganglia besides each segment of the spinal cord. But, despite intact motor nerves, Ian's brain could not coordinate any movement without knowing where his body and limbs were in space. Without peripheral feedback controlled movement was impossible. Though we are very aware of touch, and Ian remembers its absence, we are hardly aware of this sixth sense of proprioception, so deep is it within us it us, Ian had discovered for himself the effects of its loss but at this point probably did not know much more. Proprioception was first described by Charles Bell, a Scottish physiologist, anatomist, and artist:

> We use our limbs without being conscious, or at least, without any conception of the thousand parts which must conform to a single act. . . . We awake with a knowledge of the position of our limbs; this cannot be from a recollection of the action which placed them where they are; it must therefore, be a consciousness of their present condition.
>
> When a blind man, or a man with his eyes shut, stands upright . . . by what means is it that he maintains an erect position? It is obvious that he has a sense by which he knows the inclination of his body.
>
> It can only be by the adjustment of muscles that the limbs are stiffened. There is no source of knowledge but a sense of the degree of exertion in his muscular frame. . . .
>
> In truth we stand by so fine an exercise of this power, and the muscles are, from habit, directed with so much precision and with an effort so slight, that we do not know how he stand.[1]

The autoimmune attack spared the nerves of the head and face (the numbness in his mouth recovered over the next few weeks), suggesting that the surface markers recognized by the antibody were only expressed on the touch and proprioceptive nerve cells below the neck. It was not surprising that the doctors did not understand what was happening since the syndrome, now called acute sensory neuronopathy syndrome, was only described several years later.[2]

All this was in the future; for now Ian hung on as best he could. Unable to move or feel, he needed help with everything—eating, dressing, going to the toilet; it was depressing, bewildering, and humiliating for a young man of 19 who'd never been ill before. Nights were the worst, lying there awake trying to work out what was happening to him.

After 3 weeks some hope arrived as he was transferred to the Wessex Neurological Centre at Southampton. The journey, however, was a nightmare. He was propped up in the back of an ambulance with his mother, Felice, and at the first corner—without any control of posture—he fell over like a ragdoll. On the plane he was propped up in a normal seat; once airborne he was sick. Throughout the journey he was terrified of falling.

The doctors at Southampton were more knowledgeable, but this did not translate into treatment or a clear diagnosis. After a few weeks of tests, being an exhibit for medical students, and some physical therapy, it became increasingly clear that there was nothing to be done. Ian was discharged home to his parents, and to a single downstairs room with a commode.

It was the worst of times. "At home, safe only when lying down, I knew nothing about my condition and the doctors had given up, I was on the scrapheap." He could do nothing except bellow, and the only person listening was his poor mother. Felice was under a lot of pressure herself. Not only had she given up her job to look after Ian, but her older son's marriage was breaking up, and she herself had been planning to leave Ian's father before all this happened. One of her friends remembered how good she was, "I would have left home myself." Ian's friends came round to ask what was wrong and he could not answer, so he just told them to leave. He had a girlfriend whom he also finished with, telling her to find someone else. At one hospital follow-up Ian was wheeled out into the corridor while Felice stayed behind. Ian thought, "He'll be telling the old sausage the worst now." Sure enough she came out in tears, having been told Ian would be in a wheelchair for the rest of his life. But they never discussed it between themselves. Ian was determined to give it a go, and his mother equally determined to help. Though depressed he was not defeated.

Over the next few months, he found that if he looked at his arm or hand as he moved it, and concentrated on what he did, he could begin to coordinate movement. After several weeks he could put something in his mouth:

> I concentrated on moving the arm, bending the elbow and then the wrist, clenching my fingers tightly all the time round what I wanted to eat. My other arm would lift off the bed by itself and float aimlessly. Why? How could I control it, and more importantly, why should it need to be controlled? It had looked after itself before, why couldn't it now?

Reading books, he often dropped them or turned over random numbers of pages. He was passionate about jigsaw puzzles, with the main puzzle being how to pick up each piece rather than which piece went where. He preferred to feed himself than be fed, and so would spend hours with cold food rather than accept help. He learned to dress, even if it took 20 minutes to put on a sock. He refused to use a wheelchair, would not go out, and discouraged anyone from coming to see him like this.[3] He learned to "bum" his way round, sitting on his bottom with legs in front of him. At night, too frightened of failure to tell anyone, he would roll out blankets on the floor and try to walk on his knees, stomping round his room while his parents slept.

Slowly, he realized that he could only rail and shout for so long before the anger consumed him. An old school friend dropped by and asked Ian how he was getting on. He told her how frustrated he was that the doctors could not tell him much. "Why then," she replied, "be so negative?" Though she knew nothing of his case and her logic was questionable, maybe, he thought, she might be right. With the knee stomping, the feeding, and the jigsaws he began to see a way. One bright spot was his regular outpatient physiotherapy. He had a laugh with the ambulance crews that took him; one time he arranged for them to fit his limbs with air splints and explain to Felice that there had been an accident. Ian was wheeled into the house covered in splints. She was terrified, then angry at having been set up, and finally delighted that her mischievous son was back. He also enjoyed the sessions with the attractive young physiotherapists. They, in turn, saw that 3 hours a week was not enough and suggested intense inpatient rehabilitation at the regional centre in Odstock just outside Salisbury. He grabbed it.

The admitting doctor, Ted Cantrell, remembered that Ian, "showed two levels; superficially jokey but very soon you saw profound unhappiness. His family was broken and he was depressed. He had left school early because he couldn't stand it and now the only job he wanted was closed to him." Ted reckoned that Ian might, at best, do a limited desk job from a wheelchair. Fortunately he did not tell Ian that.

Ian stayed for 17 months. Every day, single-mindedly, he watched and thought his way back to movement and independence. The therapists had little understanding of his condition and his needs, but they gave him time, space, and encouragement. They thought he was improving because the neuropathy was getting better, when it was rather because of his own efforts in learning to manage. They tested him by putting different shaped objects in his hands and asked him, eyes shut, to say which was which. Not for the last time he succeeded by cheating, knowing that they made different sounds when rubbed or crushed in the hand; the star shape was painful when gripped tight. Learning to outwit the condition was the beginning of a more positive approach, learning to live with what he had rather than mourning what had been lost. He learned to draw and then to write (with completely different hand-writing); he would thread a paper clip chain for hours on end to learn how to use his fingers. But most of all he learned to stand, and in doing so became aware of the physics of movement; for every action there is a reaction. If he put one arm out, whether standing or sitting, he had to manage cognitively and brace himself and balance with the other arm, or he would fall. Every movement, every lift, had to be assessed for its consequences for his posture and safety. After 12 months he could stand and after 14 months walk unaided. Slow, laborious, and ungainly, he had reinvented the act of walking: "You cannot imagine the satisfaction derived from the simple task of being able to walk to the toilet unaided, and not be reliant upon the availability of others."

As he learned movements, he realized the very concept of "learning" had changed. When we learn a new movement, say driving, we have to concentrate as we improve, but then the movement becomes automatic and requires less thought as it becomes a skill. This never happened for Ian. Each time he had to think about it, so as his repertoire increased, the more he had to think. "The need to concentrate was (and is) total. I cannot emphasize enough the effort needed to build up in my mind every move and counter move." If he had a head cold and could not think straight, then he could not move safely.

Ted had initially put Ian in his own room, but to encourage him to make friends they moved him to the bigger ward. Within a few weeks they may have regretted it since Ian soon became ringleader of the naughty squad. Once, a man was imprisoned inside a vaulting horse in the gym. The physiotherapist returned to find smoke rings emerging from the horse. She immediately blamed Ian.

While Ian was exploring wall bars and cold food, paper clips, and cheek, Ted Cantrell was considering the next move, since he could not go back to butchery. Ian had no qualifications, so Ted suggested a course at the local college. Ian, having escaped school once, was not keen, but had little choice. He began with English, history, and sociology, but soon dropped the last two. Initially he was driven there and back each weekday, but he wanted his own wheels. At that time "the disabled" were offered appalling "invalid carriages," flimsy three-wheeled death traps, some with a small electric motor. Ian learned to drive in one of these, but they were not fast and one day he was overtaken going up a hill by a woman walking with a pram. Soon after, he was upgraded to a petrol-engined version.

After 17 months he left Odstock to spend a year at a special college for those with special physical needs, he combined studying with misbehaving. He would organize trips to pubs with a long line of invalid carriages snaking along country lanes, with him at the back as shotgun. He even managed an affair with an older women care assistant. Everyone knew, and the other students were delighted that the principal, despite his best efforts, never caught them at it. Once released from education, he found a job in the Civil Service. If anyone asked about his problem he would either have a stab at explaining or just say it was his back. His first major purchase was a proper car. A brother remarked that when Ian had the three-wheeler people would ask how he was, but with the car no-one bothered any more. With a simple hand-controlled lever in the car, up for go, down for stop, Ian passed his driving test. Against expectations, he had left the disabled world largely behind.

But life was not all work, and when he was asked to help form a group to assist newly young disabled adults he did not think twice. There he met a young woman, Mavis, who had contracted polio as a child, leaving her with a curvature of the spine and severe weakness. They fell in love and within 6 weeks Ian had proposed.

Mavis had been disabled far longer than Ian and taught him a huge amount. Ian had clawed his way to independence, single-mindedly reducing any sign of his condition. Mavis was not impressed. So now he was independent, she said, what was he going to do with it? Life was not about proving people wrong, but for living, enjoying; for savoring. She had had years of operations, hospital confinement, and missed fun; now was the time to live. They married, bought a sensible, small flat, tired of it rapidly, so bought a bungalow with a garden, did it up, and kept chickens.

For the next 6 years Ian and Mavis enjoyed work and married life, relishing their independence and each other. But then she fell ill with abdominal cramps followed by severe bleeding. They thought initially it was a spontaneous abortion and both were devastated. Further investigation confirmed that Mavis had indeed been pregnant, with twins, but that the underlying cause was advanced ovarian cancer. Within a few months she was dead, and Ian buried her on their wedding anniversary. He sold the bungalow and moved into a stark, anonymous flat, healing his wounds as best he could.

It was not long after Mavis died, and a full 12 years since the diarrhea, that at a neurological appointment he saw a young research fellow who wondered if Ian would mind doing a short test. Jonathan Cole introduced himself and explained the experiment, and then asked Ian about his condition; what was it like to live without touch and proprioception. Previous doctors had never asked. Ian did the test and was happy when Jonathan asked if he would come again for some more experiments. After 12 years Ian felt he had found a doctor who might listen, and maybe understand:

> We are social beings, whenever we experience an ailment or illness there is much comfort and solace to be gained from this "shared experience." However, the uniqueness of my disability imposed a journey that is essentially solitary. Jonathan was a breath of fresh air.

For his part Jonathan had never seen, nor imagined, a condition where a person might have a complete loss of touch and position sense with perfectly preserved pain and temperature perception and normal motor nerves. If such a person might exist, then the idea that they would stand, walk, drive, and live independently was astonishing. The only similar case he knew of was described by John Rothwell and colleagues in London.[4] Their subject had a severe sensory neuropathy that had affected the distal parts of his limbs and spared the motor fibers. In laboratory tests they showed that he was able to do certain tasks, such a make a figure of eight in the air, but despite this, his hands were relatively useless to him in daily life. He could not hold a pen or write, nor fasten his shirt buttons or hold a cup in one hand, and he lived from a wheelchair. How could Ian manage so much? Jonathan needed more time to think. Over the next few months they met several times as Jonathan devised experiments to confirm Ian's sensory loss and to explore his movement ability.

Ian's introduction to neuroscience was neither exotic nor pleasurable. Jonathan had to prove, as best he could, the absence of the nerves underpinning touch and proprioception. This was done through clinical neurophysiological tests involving stimulating and recording from nerves in the arms and legs. Soaked felt pad electrodes were placed over the peripheral nerves, say at the wrist or ankle, and similar recording electrodes positioned over a muscle in the hand or foot for a movement or motor nerve, or over the same nerve further up the limb for a sensory response. A small electric current was passed through the skin to activate the nerve at one site, and the resulting impulses recorded from the muscle or nerve at another. This is usually slightly unpleasant rather than painful and is tolerated well:

> I love it when doctors say, "This isn't going to hurt." I remember vividly during my early days at the Neuro Centre there was a very painful test with a circular clip attached to my fingers. I said it hurt, they said it didn't; the red, sore rings around my fingers supported me. So you can imagine my skepticism when being approach to being a guinea pig. But my trust in Jonathan began during those early tests.

Peripheral nerves contain various classes of nerve cell or axon. The largest are the movement or motor nerves starting in the spinal cord and going to muscles. The next largest are sensory nerves which underpin the sensations of touch and movement sense, designated A-beta cells. The nerve cells in both of these classes are wrapped in a sheath of insulating tissue, myelin, which allows them to conduct faster, at around 50 m/s. The next type is smaller myelinated sensory fibers conducting at 12–20 m/s; these A-delta fibers relay impulses underpinning the perceptions of sharp pain and warmth. The smallest fibers, C fibers, are not myelinated and conduct impulses perceived as duller pain and warmth at 0.5–2 m/s or so. Because of the properties of these nerve cells the large ones are excited at low intensities by electrical stimuli through the skin, but to excite the smaller ones the current has to be higher and becomes painful, so these are not stimulated in clinical practice. The tests also involve placing small needle electrodes through the skin into muscles, electromyography (EMG), which confirms that the motor nerves are all intact.

Ian's studies showed normal movement or motor nerve results, and normal EMG, with a complete absence of A-beta sensory nerve responses. This supported Ian's loss of touch and movement/position sense with preserved power. Moreover, at intensities at which control subjects perceive the electrical shock and even at intensities beginning to be felt as unpleasant, Ian felt nothing. The large sensory nerves were gone.

Next Jonathan planned further tests with a friend and colleague in Southampton, Haider Katifi, to see if there was any evidence of sensory nerve function from recording over the sensory cortex, using electrodes on the scalp. The cortex acts like an amplifier; perhaps a small cortical response might be recorded from stimulating a nerve that might be missed from recording peripherally. No cortical evoked potentials were found. As well as Ian's lack of perception of touch and movement sensation, they also found no peripheral or cortical evoked potentials from the brain. There was no demonstrable A-beta sensory nerve-mediated activity.[5]

As they experimented and chatted, Jonathan was fascinated to see how controlled Ian's movements were. People with sensory loss were supposed to move with uncertain, shaking movements, known as ataxia, and yet he was smooth and solid. Jonathan tested this by asking Ian to hold down a typewriter key connected to a strain gauge and measuring his stability. Without seeing what he was doing, Ian could maintain a very small force for several minutes, in contrast to the subject investigated by John Rothwell, who soon lost control. He seemed to be able to maintain a force output without knowing what it was.[6] But when Ian was asked to match such a force in one hand by pressing down another key using a finger from the other hand he could not.

People who have lost a limb are still aware of the limb and sometimes feel it moving, a phenomenon called phantom limb sensation. This is thought to be due to there being a signal within the brain, associated with the command to move, which can be perceived. Ian had no phantom limb sensation, nor any feeling when a limb was moved by others, and no feeling when he made a movement himself. Jonathan, this time with another friend, Louis Merton, used a technique called transcranial magnetic stimulation (TMS) to activate Ian's motor cortex cells in the brain (painlessly) to cause a small twitch movement of the arm.[7] With his eyes shut Ian had no awareness of this. So, just as he had no perception of his own motor command, so an artificially induced movement led to no percept either. So, he had no phantom sensation and no central awareness of his own or an artificially induced sensory correlate of a motor command. Maybe Ian's had faded without reinforcement from the moving limb or body.

In another TMS experiment Jonathan, with Louis, asked Ian to make a small movement of either his thumb or first finger every second. Then, when this was established as a rhythm, just before a movement, Jonathan superimposed a small TMS pulse. Now TMS, at high intensities, leads to painless muscle twitches by activating the motor cortex cells by a pulse of depolarization, which in turn makes the muscles twitch. At low intensities, as used here, no twitch is seen when the subject is at rest. But, as a subject begins to will a movement, that act leads to cells in the motor cortex becoming ready to fire by their resting membrane potentials falling. Then the effect of the intention to act, summed with a small TMS current, leads to a small twitch in only those muscles the subject is thinking of activating. In other words, by looking at twitches seen at sub-threshold levels for a TMS twitch at rest, they reasoned that they were able to look at the focus of intention to move, or the motor command.

They recorded from several muscles over the hand and forearm to see the intensity of TMS needed to activate those muscles when they were partially primed during the intention to move. In control subjects any intention to move the thumb led to small TMS-induced twitches in the thumb muscle, but also to twitches in other muscles in the hand and forearm. This makes sense, since most natural movements involve the whole hand and not just one finger joint. But when Ian was asked to move his thumb, small TMS-induced movements were only seen in the thumb muscle. In other words he had learned how to move in a different way, with focused intention on the target muscle alone. Ian's movements might look like ours, but this experiment had shown that his attention and thinking had led to very different activation patterns in Ian's motor cortex.[8]

In parallel with these experiments, Ian and Jonathan started talking about Ian's life since the neuronopathy. Jonathan wanted to know how Ian had thought (and fought) his way back to movement and how he managed from day to day. Over the next few months Jonathan learned as much by talking with Ian as he did in the lab. He began to realize that there were two ways to understand how someone lives without the sensations of touch and proprioception, one involving experiments and the other by listening to Ian. Jonathan was how amazed by Ian's extraordinary response to his condition and asked Ian if he might write his biography. Ian agreed, and *Pride and a Daily Marathon* was born. Its title arose from Ian's sheer, relentless bloody pride and arrogance (Felice's words) without which he might never have recovered, and "the daily marathon" came from Ian himself. One day, trying to explain the mental effort he needed to move, he'd likened it to running a marathon every day.

Despite all this activity Ian did not become a full-time subject. At work in the statistical office he was promoted more than once and he also met a girl called Linda. They became a couple, though Ian was reluctant to commit again. Linda bided her time, waited for a leap year and asked him to marry her one February 29th. They married that summer in a beautiful old chapel within the Roman fort at Portchester Castle. Then, tired of the office, they moved north to the English Lakes to start their new life. *Pride* ended with Ian and Linda heading into a Lakeland sunset hand in hand.

Pride and a Daily Marathon was completed in 1989 and published 2 years later. It detailed Ian's condition and his response to it, a single-minded focus on returning to a "normal" life, with everything second to that. Overall it was a story of triumph and unexpected functional recovery, similar to some accounts of impairment in the popular press, in which the person takes on and triumphs over their problem; what Ian calls the "one legged man climbs Everest" approach.[9]

Since then much has happened in his life; there have been many experiments, but perhaps more importantly has been time for him to explore his condition more deeply. In retrospect the busy years between illness and *Pride* were insufficient for Ian to go beyond the triumph/tragedy models of disability to the infinitely more subtle and complex reconciliation with his condition which he now shows. Today he lives from a wheelchair, mainly because of back problems but also because he is more at peace with his condition and its demands on him. Not standing frees time and mental effort for other things. Reconciled to his condition, he has earned his living for many years as a consultant on disability issues, specializing in accessibility in the built environment, using the demands of his disability—attention to movement and to his immediate environment—to his advantage. He has moved from wanting to appear non-disabled to living with his condition, and he is one of the more effective and quiet advocates within the disability community. This transition is reflected within the new account.

Ian's life has never been dull and there is much to tell about the last 25 years. Among many other episodes, he has become an expert in two widely different areas, disability access audit and rare varieties of turkeys, collaborated on a TV documentary and two theatre plays, and made numerous trips including to NASA and a flight into zero gravity. He has met several other people with similar conditions, if not similar recovery in movement, and swopped notes.

One day Ian was musing on a title for this account and suggested, among others, "Guinea Pig's Tale," reflecting his thoughts on being a long-term participant in experiments. Though *Pride* contained some neuroscience, it was early days. Since then Ian has visited labs in the UK, Europe, and the USA as scientists have designed experiments to understand his condition and his exploration of the limits of movement without peripheral feedback. Of course there are many subjects with unusual conditions who have generously given their time to research, but arguably none has been in a position to tell what it is like to be a subject quite like Ian. Further, he is not content to be passive, and increasingly makes suggestions during experiments and holds strong views on some labs and their approaches. So here Ian shares some of his thoughts on neuroscience and, ominously, on neuroscientists. The account, however, does not detail lab visits and experiments laboriously, but rather focuses on those visits which altered Ian's views of his condition or which revealed particularly interesting facets of it.[10]

Chapter 1, "Like Breathing," follows Ian and Linda as they settle in the Lakes and renovate their house. While she worked, Ian took time out. But he could not be idle (comparatively—his condition prevents that in any case) and he soon explored an idea to write guides for disabled people visiting tourist sites and hotels. Taking its cue from his handiwork at home, the chapter ends with Ian's thoughts on the relations between thought and action and how immersed he can be in what he does.

There follow two chapters on visits to foreign laboratories. "Z-axis and the Tombstone" relates how Ian travelled to Munich and Hamburg to visit two very different workers, one interested in the awareness of whole-body orientation in space and the other in the mechanisms of pain perception. The experiments were complex, with painful or disorientating protocols. On returning from Germany Ian cooperated with some rather more sedate research in Oxford and was a guest at High Table in Christ Church. The chapter discloses one reason why he was prepared to cooperate in research which was, at times, an ordeal. But perhaps the main revelation was less what he did than how he remembers it. His memories of going to Germany are startlingly detailed and completely unlike other people's.

His next trips were to Quebec and to Marseilles, hence "French Connections." In addition to research, he also met Ginette Lizotte, a Québécois woman who is one of the few people in the world with a similar condition. Their meeting, and Ian's reactions to it, bring some of his actions into question. The chapter details some of the research, but also the start of his journey from being a passive subject to questioning the science and the scientists.

Soon after he returned from Canada he moved back down south to the New Forest. In "Hungry" we follow him during a wretched time as he starts over yet again. Through his own hard work and effort he begins to find a new paid career as a disability access audit consultant.

There follow two chapters in which Ian and neuroscience meet showbiz. In "*L'Homme Qui*" Ian reflects on his life being represented as one of the vignettes in Peter Brook's play of the same name that toured France, the UK, Europe, and the USA. The other studies were based around cases found in Oliver Sacks' *The Man Who Mistook His Wife for a Hat*. Ian's vignette was the only one drawn directly from a single person, and indeed from talking to and observing Ian at first hand when he went to Paris to assist Peter and his ensemble. How did it feel to Ian to sit in The National Theatre, London and watch a professional actor portray him on stage?

The next chapter details Ian portraying himself in a BBC *Horizon* documentary, "The Man Who Lost His Body."[11] He lost his anonymity but brought insights into proprioception and the consequences of its loss to millions of people round the world in a way which no number of scientific papers ever could.

Being disabled is boring, and having a condition which imposes on every second of one's waking life even more so. The play and program were both fun and also validated his extraordinary response to his condition through the interest and fascination of Brook, actors, the TV crew, and the BBC. But fun could also be had from science. The next chapter, "Going Parabolic: the Pull of Zero Gravity," follows Ian to Boston and then to NASA in Houston as he flies in zero gravity aboard the "Vomit Comet." Ian would rarely volunteer to place himself in such an extreme environment, but this was too great an opportunity to turn down. "Perfect Day" returns to Ian's home life. In a few years he founds his own company, moves house twice, becomes a national expert on turkeys, and remarries.

Much of the science has looked at how Ian moves and the limits to movement without feedback. In contrast Chapters 9 and 10 detail work which comes closer to revealing something of his core sense of self. "Throwaways: Gesture in Chicago" details the work of David McNeill in Chicago on Ian's gesture and how he has managed to embody feeling and expression with language. Ian is both critical and admiring of this work, and unafraid to debate with David. McNeill's studies with Ian have allowed him to extend his theory of gesture. David describes, in language unusual for a scientist, how exciting it was to see Ian's gestures and speech, "As if we were touching the origin of language."

Another series of experiments with Ian and Ginette looked at a novel class of peripheral nerve and cutaneous receptors which appear to have a role in the perception of the pleasantness of silk on the skin or of a light caress. Since Ian and Ginette no longer possess the main myelinated nerves underpinning light touch, the perceptual feeling of CT nerve activations can be studied in them, and only them. "Feeling the Warmth" begins with a consideration of Ian's and Ginette's roles in the scientific investigation of these nerves but is then extended to approach Ian's residual cutaneous perception in relation to intimacy. A measure of how far Ian has travelled since becoming ill, how curious he is about his condition, and just how sophisticated his analysis of his own functioning has become lies within these two chapters in which he collaborates with neuroscience exploring the boundaries between the neuronopathy and his embodied self.

In the last chapter, "Nothing Lost," Ian reflects on his condition 40 years on and describes why he ever collaborated in scientific and biographical work. He gives his views on the different sorts of science he has seen and discusses meeting famous people like Peter Brook and Oliver Sacks. Ian's response to his sensory loss and his performances in experiments and his daily activities have always impressed; so much so that some have wondered how much automaticity, or even neurological recovery, might have occurred. In turn, he has been his own worst enemy in that he will never allow himself to be seen when not at his best. In an extended section, he describes what happened when the lights went out at home when he was on his own. However much he has improved, the condition's hold is as severe as ever. Appropriately the final words come from Herb Schaumburg, one of Ian's favorite scientists and the man who first described Ian's condition.

One of the most famous subjects in neuroscience, HM, who lost memory following neurosurgery for epilepsy, once mused that, "We live and learn. I live, you learn."[12] It has always been a concern that Ian might feel more was being taken than given. In "Nothing Lost," though, he describes how the science, the lectures, the travel, and the TV and theater have enriched his life in ways he would not otherwise have imagined.

In *Pride* Jonathan made a minimal appearance. Since then, however, he has been involved so much in the science that it was not possible to keep him out of this volume completely. But he was concerned to be as small a presence as possible and to avoid his friendship with Ian over 30 years coloring the account. Having said that, he felt he should write something about Ian from his own perspective, and so in a short Afterword he has combined this with some of the memories of Ian from some the scientists, artists, choreographers, magicians, and philosophers he has worked with and who have enjoyed—and are enjoying—collaborating with him thus far.

When he and Jonathan first met it was 12 years after the onset of Ian's neuronopathy; now it is over 40. *Pride* detailed a young man's "triumph" over disability with little of the science of deafferentation. The present account is a more mature and complete reflection. Though it shows how he has turned impairment to his advantage (in his work in disability access audit), and how it has altered the ways in which he sees the world, "triumph over" has been replaced by an infinitely richer and deeper "coming to terms with." Now, in his 60s, Ian has the whole new challenge of living with such a demanding condition as he ages.

The five chapters on science, as he travels round the world, feature only a small part of the empirical work he has assisted with. Rather than detail each laboratory and experiment, these chapters also follow Ian's scientific education as he moves from "guinea pig," to participant, assistant, and critic. The book questions the very idea of Ian as passive participant to show how he is actively involved in experiments; one never does an experiment *on* him but always *with* him. His first-person account of the experience and strategies employed are crucial to interpretation of the third-person results. But he goes beyond even these to reveal himself as a cogent and insightful critic of neuroscience itself.

The book details neuroscience, art, documentary, and biography. Each is required and all are complimentary. As one senior neuroscientist says, in addition to experimentation, Ian showed that "to understand a particular experience is, first-person testimony from people who live with that experience is the best bet." At its heart, then, is a fusion of narrative and neuroscience, of the personal and the physiological, to understand touch and proprioception and its loss, and Ian Waterman's extraordinary response to his impairment.

1

LIKE BREATHING

It is an old cliché, but I was the first disabled person I knew. I wasn't that impressed at the time. I just thought I had to work hard to be normal, well at least to *appear* normal. Society is far more accepting now, but back then, 30 years ago and more, I knew I had to look after and manage myself. If I stayed as bad as I was in the first year or so then life would be pretty grim, in part because of the impact on my parents and family. That was a big driving force, in fact the biggest.

Forty years later, there are still times when Ian feels awkward, for instance when walking and he looks different. Sometimes he can cope with the stares, sometimes not. After the death of his first wife, Mavis, he became independent and solitary. He would occasionally turn up at a supermarket but not go inside to avoid being stared at by children, or because he knew he might fumble for change, or sometimes simply because he did not have the energy. If he backed out then he would be critical of himself for ages. Slowly, though, he accepted that everyone can have a bad day, so why could he not too? Just as an athlete cannot run at his or her best every day, so he could not function near maximum the whole time. Though he became more accommodating, he remained, and remains, hard on himself:

> I would not go out, except on my terms. I did not go to weddings, did not go to social events, unless on my terms. I managed my life and my mobility, but I had created and become a bit of a monster.[1] That may appear harsh, but it was necessary. Without being that monster I would not have survived.

In hospital, before learning to stand and walk, he would not go out in a wheelchair. For all his apparent "bloody mindedness," people did not understand what Ian was coping with. His brothers, for instance, had no idea of his disability and its impact. They realized that Ian needed to have lights on the whole time, but not the effort involved in movement, in appearing "normal."[2] *Pride and a Daily Marathon* helped a little; one brother said how sorry he was; he had had no idea what Ian had been through before reading it.

Ian has now come more to terms with the condition and can leave the monster behind, at least a little. But this is not to say that he finds his level of everyday functioning easy. He talks of "downtime;" he puts so much concentration and effort into everything that he needs a break, either with a coffee and snack for a few minutes during the day, in a secure seat, or—better—a bed on which he just flops. Then—and only then—when he does not have to think about posture and movement, can he relax.[3] One friend asked him if, when he got home in the evening, he made himself a gin and tonic and chilled out. "But," Ian replied, "sitting is a task I think about and the glass is fragile and I have to grip it so carefully to avoid it slipping or breaking."[4] Relaxation means no concentration on movement. In addition to short periods of downtime, Ian also needs days off; days when he does not have to push himself, days without constant thought about movement and its prediction and consequences.

Sometimes though, Ian needs a longer break; a sabbatical from work altogether. By the end of his time in the Civil Service he was not sleeping. He was doing the job well enough and had been promoted, but it was taking its toll, due less to the work than to the requirements for movement. Each day he had to move round the office, go to meetings, often while carrying something and having a conversation. He would come home exhausted and unable to turn off:

> Mavis would come home from a busy day with the police around midnight, and she would take an hour to settle down. It was like that for me, running over a meeting or the work I had done, not so much rerunning the "work" elements, rather thinking about my movements. Operating at such a pitch it took a while to wind down. Maybe that is why actors or rock stars do drugs, to come down. Taking an afternoon off did not do it. I needed to completely unwind. I needed weeks not hours. And even a holiday involving movement would present problems. A real holiday is a holiday from thinking about movement, sitting in a chair looking at a movie or reading a book.

Where possible he would also mentally rehearse the next day for its physical moves, like a dancer.[5] So, throughout the last three decades, he has had long periods off to relax and recharge:

> Sitting in the forest cradled by the roots of a tree, listening to the wind overhead, with no thoughts, just being there; that's as close as it gets to heaven for me. I once drifted off and awoke to a dusting of snow ... Wow. Then reality kicked in, how the hell was I going to get back to the car?

Once married, he and his second wife, Linda, left the Civil Service and moved 300 miles north to the Lake District, an area of mountains and peace. He had worked for 12 years and earned promotions, all the time laughing his problem off as a bad back. He needed time with Linda, and time out from work. It was a big move; he had always lived on the south coast, between Southampton and Portsmouth, all his friends and family were around and his beloved New Forest was just along the motorway. Once in the Lakes he realized just how exhausted he was. The plan was for Linda to work and he would take time out for a while. They would find their feet and then open a bed and breakfast place accessible for people with impairment and their families and/or carers. Linda was a fine cook, especially of cakes and pastries, and was itching to use her skills professionally. They took a gamble since Ian was leaving work and Linda took a pay cut, but they thought it worth the risk.

They moved during the recession of the 1980s and found that their house down south did not sell; so, unable to buy, they rented a barn in Kendal. The views were spectacular, though it was a shame it leaked so much and that mushrooms grew on the window sill. It was also isolated down a dirt track, which was far from ideal for Ian. After 6 months a friend of Linda's from work had an offer of a position in Jersey for 2 years, so they rented her cottage. It was the oldest place in a small town, Sedburgh, at the foot of the Howgill Fells.[6] Ian could never use the front steps up into the house and came and went through the back way. He pottered to the newspaper shop, the butcher, and the pub and got to know the locals.

Eventually they found their own place just outside a small village. Stainton Hall was an old farmhouse, one of a group of houses that were stretched out along a winding river. It had recently been done up, badly, and Ian set about re-doing it, stripping wallpaper, painting, and decorating. Game though he was, his rate of progress was slow and they needed to bring in plasterers, builders, and electricians. It was a drain both financially and emotionally. The house also had electrical supply problems, not ideal when Ian relied on electric lights indoors, and the river also flooded regularly, leaving them marooned on their own little island for days several times a year.

Around this time Ian first phoned Jonathan to say he was in bed with a bad back. Ian never normally complained, so Jonathan drove up to see him. They had long discussed the extra pressure Ian put on his joints and back, and he was well aware that something, sometime, might go. He was also phlegmatic; he knew he would probably not be able to maintain his mobility forever and so took each day as it came. His hatred of doctors was also as strong as ever. Jonathan pushed him into seeing his GP and then an orthopedic surgeon, thinking he had probably slipped a disk and, with his permission, wrote to both to explain Ian's problem. The surgeon was less than helpful, suggesting there was little to be done because of Ian's "condition." Fortunately it all settled down with 6 weeks in bed, though that was not the downtime Ian had hoped for.

If their choice of house was not ideal neither, a little surprisingly, was the Lake District:

> I loved the Lakes very much indeed. Living there, however, was never as successful as living near the New Forest. Though more scenic in some ways—it had the mountains and the views—it was nowhere near as accessible. We had an Airedale, a big hairy terrier, and I used to take her out every day for some exercise. Obviously I could not walk her terribly well, though she would walk with me quite well on the lead. I used to take her to an old Quaker cemetery up on the high hills, completely enclosed by a stone wall. I would park the car, and let her run in there.

It was a remote area, quiet, peaceful, and very beautiful, but Ian could not explore because the ground was too uneven. He had a knack of looking at a map and finding places which were remote and yet accessible, but in this regard the Lakes were not kind.

His passion, before going up to the Lakes, was photography. One of the ideas for going up there was to start a postcard business. But he could only get the same old views others got, and gave up that idea. He focused, instead, on macrophotography and nature; mushrooms, an early bud, or, say, lichen on a gate. He would spent days looking for an accessible car park with somewhere nearby he could walk to take photos.

Ian had planned to rest for a while, bed in, and then work. Something else, though, had been at the back of his mind. When he was in rehabilitation at Odstock Hospital the physiotherapists had been preparing a guide for disabled people who wanted to explore Salisbury. The city was only a couple of miles away so they used to take patients down there to reintroduce them to the world. They asked him if he would see how accessible the cathedral was for disabled people. Ian knew what was behind it:

> Get him out and give him some confidence, and if he fails we can always go to get him. I had not been out on my own for nearly 18 months and was being disruptive; I knew it was time to move on. The cathedral visit was to get me back into society; my first big adventure. So I got into my little car and went down several times.

Clueless about access, he wandered around trying to think up a plan. He noted down the number of steps, the length and steepness of ramps, and how easy it was to use the toilet. In the hospital he had spent his time concentrating on how to move his body, with little thought about how he would actually get around in a busy place. Before his illness, like most of us, he had moved around without thinking about the distances or steps involved. Now, in the cathedral, he began to see the built environment not as a space he could just drift through while thinking of something else, but as a place with physicality and bustle which determined his access to and enjoyment of it. He realized he would have to think ahead and plan his movement from one part of the building to another, decomposing each stretch into sections with pauses, similar to how a climber would think their way up a cliff face. Ian's walks were, from now on, horizontal ascents. "Yes, I am your Chris Bonnington of the horizontal world, although I suppose given walking is like a hyper-reality chess game, maybe I am more a Spassky."

In the vast cathedral space, plotting and planning, he became absorbed in its spaces and steps. Moving round in the hospital and at home, relearning to walk, he had focused on himself. Now, he was using his experience to frame that of others, whether with problems in movement, hearing, or vision. It took him out of himself and allowed him to get under the building's skin, to see it more deeply and clearly. After months cloistered in the ward, the real world—with real people (and real cloisters)—though risky and daunting, was alive and he relished it:

> I absolutely loved going to the cathedral after all that time incarcerated in hospital. But, wow, was it an eye opener to my situation. I went round and started to think about how people in wheelchairs might get about. I had simply never thought about that before; I had just thought about my movements all the time. But how I plan my campaign to get around a building has implications for others. My needs for a flat level surface are the same as for someone with a wheelchair, for example. But there was also this thing about access and giving information for others. Now I saw the building in a different way, as I saw the world very differently. You look at the hill and wonder if you can run up it. I look and want to see if there is a track and a car park I can use at the top. Our aim is the same but ways to do it different.

It was also fun:

> Every few minutes a verger would appear with another school group. I was making notes about a ramp when a party turned up and he said "What do we notice about all the statues in the cathedral . . . their feet are all pointing down the nave, towards the altar." About 15 minutes later another group of kids are there and the verger asks the same question. "Which way are the feet pointing?" One little girl thought for a second and said, "Up."

Back at the hospital the physiotherapists were impressed with how detailed and comprehensive his notes were. But then they knew that under the pranks and humor lay a determined and incredibly disciplined mind. He saw an educational psychologist, "a boffin asking strange questions." Some weeks later the report suggested Ian was determined, intelligent, and would do well in whatever he did.

After the cathedral he left Odstock for a year at college before working in the Civil Service for a decade. But the idea of access audit had never faded completely, and it resurfaced in the Lakes:

> I had gone full of hope, wanting to do things around access and write a guide to the Lakes for disabled people. I contacted the local freebie newspaper, run by the tourism people, and offered to write something on a regular basis about access. They were not interested, so I started compiling information for my own guide. Every couple of weeks or so I would explore somewhere and see how accessible it was.

He visited 30 or 40 attractions, and noted down what he thought would be useful; parking, how accessible the environment was, basic amenities etc. There was a stained glass gallery in Ambleside; how far was the car park, did it have accessible bays, where exactly was it located? At that time, before the internet, there was not much information for disabled people, just a few musty, outdated guides. Ian tried to interest the local paid-for newspaper. Its office was on the second floor, and not easy to get to. Nothing came of it; he was too far ahead of the game.

Existing guides were often written by the people who owned the attractions, and were unimpaired, which Ian thought was crazy. He was so angry that one place was completely different from its blurb that he phoned the Holiday Care Service, a charity concerned with providing advice about holidays for those with special needs. His call was put through to its boss, Maundy Todd. She was very impressed by Ian's passion and so came up to visit him. If he thought he could do better—and she thought he probably could—then would he like to do their work up in the north? The snag was that being a charity they could only pay expenses. Thinking this would be an opening, Ian accepted immediately.

The Holiday Care Service used a simple one-, two-, or three-star grading system but Ian thought there had to be a better way. He was no fool either; he knew that around 10% of the population were disabled, and that most of them travelled with their wives, husbands, or partners; their disposable income was considerable. Ian could see a living in this. He also knew that the government was preparing a flagship Disability Discrimination Act which was bound to create work.

His patch was from Scotland to Birmingham, a distance of 500 miles north to south. One week he surveyed 12 places round Scotland on his own, two or three a day. No one taught him, he just learned as he went, phoning Maundy if he was stuck. He always wrote more than they wanted, and it was soon clear just how good he was. Maundy was amazed:

> Why was I better? Most of the other judges were not disabled. OK, most gynecologists are men and you don't need to be disabled to audit buildings, but there are times

when it helps. When talking about distance between places and access, if you are disabled you have a better understanding. It was my grounding in access audits. There were books out there, but I thought there should be a practical way in to it. "Turn adversity to your advantage" was my mantra. I have a disability; I should try to use it.

The others were counting steps, looking at distances; ticks in the box. For me it was the whole thing. I might want to go on the terrace like everyone else; there might be steps up and the hotel people would say, "You don't need to go on the terrace." But I wanted to do everything everyone else did, why not? I wrote everything up, not just the ramps but the attitude of the owners and how that was translated into their building. I wrote up the whole experience, as it was for me, looking at the fuller picture. Since I have to be so careful in moving, I was also closer to what I was describing.

Ironically, though he was close in his need to calculate every movement and step, with little or no feel from the body he could not feel the ground or the gravel, or the wood banister, or the weight of a knife in his hand. His thoroughness was, at one level, that of an acrobat measuring distances and angles, and at another level that of an academic, thinking his way round each hotel, first as someone with a mobility problem, then as someone with a hearing impairment or visual problem. His need for intellectual immersion in actions we normally do without thought was, here at least, an advantage.

At each hotel he would introduce himself, ask if there any concerns and then do a journey through the hotel:

Can I find it? Is it easy for visually impaired people? Can I park, is it level, can I walk across, and are there ramps into the hotel? Is there egress in case of fire? Is the entrance independently accessible to a cross section of people? Do you have to interact with it to open it? Is there a button to press? Do you have to talk to someone out of hours? How well lit is it? Can the handle be opened by someone with a dexterity problem? If a glass door, then can it be seen? I don't want to walk into a pane of glass. Is the door heavy? I don't want to fall over trying to open it.

I looked at lighting, width of path, gradient, how exposed it is in the rain? For visually impaired people what is the sound of a gravel path compared with a concrete one? Is there a handrail for them to run a stick along? With partial vision are signs the right size, colors visible? I want to get to the reception and need a sign above the desk. How do you book in; can a wheelchair user do it? If hearing impaired is there loop supported hearing? You talk to the people and soon pick up if they are switched on.

I am able to put these disparate elements into context and see the accessibility of the building as a whole. The access auditing was just an extension of what I had been doing anyway. I stand outside my condition to help others, but anyway their concerns overlap with mine. Lighting is important for me. At night how do I get to an accessible parking space if there is no lighting? It is a safety issue for me and many others. If someone is not agile, it is an issue, as it is to me.

All that before he got to the hotel rooms themselves. Each hotel had its accessible rooms and it was those he focused on, together with the restaurant, bar, and public spaces. At one hotel in Blackpool the manager asked him to let him know when he audited the accessible accommodation so he could come along:

> I did the whole building except the disabled room and then went back to pick up the manager. We got the lift to the second floor. The corridor was long and narrow and the room half way along. It was a fairly well done accessible bedroom with a twin bed and an OK bathroom.
>
> I asked who had designed it. He was obviously pleased with it and said they had a local architect in. I asked about his background in disability. He had none, but had had words with the manager's disabled nephew and worked it round that. And I said the nephew would be around 12, because everything was geared to the dimensions of a child. I explained that adults in wheelchairs have a different height range and he got quite irate. "But we've just spent thousands of pounds on this." I said I cannot pass it as being accessible since it does not meet the requirements. He got very angry but I could not help it.

When things calmed down a bit Ian asked another question.

> "Why did you choose this room?" The manager replied, "Because it has the best view. Why?" The problem was that you could not get a wheelchair down the narrow corridor and in through the door; you couldn't do a right angle turn into it. He just lost the plot and got very angry. He had done it all with the best of intent, but had wasted his money. It was not accessible.

Later that same day, Ian looked at another hotel whose owner had been really grumpy over the phone. When Ian walked in the owner said, "You're disabled; good. We get all these people coming round telling us what to do and they haven't got a clue. I have always said they should get disabled people to do it. All they say is, 'Make it white, make it that height . . .' but it's never a disabled person. . . ." Ian went round, and though it was poorly done he gave some advice and the owner was happy.

Even now, 30 years later, Ian can still remember almost every hotel he has audited or been in. It is second nature for him to absorb the details of accessibility:

> I could walk them all in my mind. I am there, imagining the place; as you could go through the lobby, to the left there are seats and to the right is the breakfast area and beyond that are the meeting rooms and there is an accessible toilet there. Three meeting rooms out to the side and one other at angles. I might miss a step somewhere but I would not miss a big issue. One in Chester has an accessible bedroom, but the restaurant is on the first floor with no lift. So they advertise themselves as accessible but if you are disabled you can't eat with the others.

Am I better at this because of my disability? Absolutely not. It is like people who are blind, they aren't fitted with hypersensitive fingers. They just attend more to what they are touching, and it is the same with me in the built environment, I attend more.

In between audit trips he worked at home, wall-papering and hacking at brambles and nettles. He was slow but enjoyed it. The quality of that enjoyment is, however, different. People enjoy walking or running, for the scenery but also for the physical joy of making and feeling their body move, lost in the movement.[7] It is never like that for Ian:

I don't get lost in walking; I concentrate all the way through. I concentrate standing up scraping wall paper, if I day dream I would fall over. I get satisfaction at the end of the job, to think "I did that." I wouldn't say I enjoy it when doing it. You may get satisfaction from running and enjoying it, during it. For me it would be satisfaction at having finished in a certain time and having pushed myself. It's a challenge; did I meet it?

If there was no satisfaction in moving, then did he enjoy constructing ideas for movement in his head, working out how to do something?

In the early days I would often plan the day in my head first. I would run through, say, a long queue for a taxi. After a long day, I would collapse not from the physical side but from the mental strain. My satisfaction is that I did it, not in constructing the movement. Once I had learned my basic alphabet of movements I would just juggle them in different ways. When I was a child in Jersey I remember going bait digging and jumping on the rocks. I used to run for the school at cross-country and remember that vividly too. I know what you are getting at; I used to enjoy the physicality of running and jumping, I do not get that anymore.

I get some pleasure at the challenge, but never the same feeling of satisfaction from movement. Cutting brambles I cannot be lost in the movement; I'd fall over. Life is more structured, cognitive. The life lived is in the head, which makes you insular and remote and maybe less approachable.

Though not in the moment, I always have to be aware of the moment I am in. When walking I have to think far ahead. But I do get absorbed in all sorts of things. If I get involved in photography I cut everything else out. Once I was peering through the lens and suddenly had a lot of sky in the picture, and only then did I realize that I was falling backwards. My prime consideration has to be safety. I can only be absorbed when completely safe.

Audit work is a satisfying blend of his needs transposed to those of others. "Yes, it can be very satisfying and it flows out of how I move round a building. It was a natural step to write about it." Though he cannot become absorbed in his own movement, he does love to see grace in others. He used to go to a deer sanctuary in the New Forest, for the peace but also to admire the grace of the animals, and enjoys sport and dance for the precision and beauty of movement.

It is curious that Ian found such energy and enthusiasm for audit and decorating, and for all the other things, when he had gone to the Lakes for rest and a respite from work. But, for him, there is a huge difference between movements imposed on him by a job and those he initiates himself:

> If I do an access audit, I know when I will do it. I might do a hotel or two in a day and then get back exhausted. But I would do it in my own time, managing myself. Then I can do another next day, feeling fresh again. In contrast, with a nine to five job, I have to perform, arrive on time, work appropriately, attend a meeting, go somewhere, do something physical; a framework I do not control. Even being sedentary at a desk you still have to get there and move and talk and go in lifts, it all builds up to make it very difficult to manage. When others are dictating there is no time frame you can control.

He needed to manage his time and energy. It might be just as arduous, but it unfurled in a way he could control. At the end he might be tired, but it was *his* tiredness. "I could not go back to a nine to five. I'd be back to where I was before the Lakes. It would absolutely exhaust me."

During his time in Odstock he had focused on escape; both from hospital and from appearing disabled. Now, with this access work, he had returned to the disability arena, 10 years or so later. But Ian did not see it quite like that. Even at Odstock, working so hard to appear normal, he was mindful of the needs of those with other impairments:

> They opened a swimming pool for patients. Some guys in chairs could not get to the changing rooms because the doors were not wide enough. I was really angry and complained. I was half way there to thinking about access. After the cathedral I had not fully seen it, but in the Lakes I realized I could do it, and maybe make a living.
>
> It was easy to put myself in others' situations. How can I place myself in the position of someone in a wheelchair when I fought so hard to get out of one? It is not rocket science. They need wide access and level floors. I like those things too. I am looking for easy routes in, shallow ramps, easy doors; my needs are the same as wheelchair users'. More difficult is thinking about visual impairments. I had friends like that and going out with them you begin to understand their needs. If in a pub and they ask where the toilet is, you might say it's down there on the right. But they need more precise instructions, so they need distance, and the colour of the door. Being in their company allows you to pick up their requirements. I also bumped into people with disabilities in college and learned a lot. My disability is a fact of life; I accept it and, indeed, I used it to my advantage for audits.

Access is not just a job for Ian, or even a passion, it is part of who he is. As a child and young man, a runner and sportsman, he was fascinated by movement in all its forms. Now the fascination continues, differently and more deeply:

> I am fascinated by the choreography of people in space. I love to observe how people move in buildings. Architects should sit and watch how people get through buildings. If they did then things might change. It is my life-blood. I just cannot go into a building, hospital, or hotel and not think whether it meets a broad spectrum of disabled people's needs. I just cannot turn it off, it is like breathing.[8]

Z-AXIS AND THE TOMBSTONE

As research papers involving Ian were published, so he was invited to visit other labs. The first two invitations to come from abroad were from Germany; one interested in the alteration of touch sensation after a type of bee sting and the other in his awareness of whole-body position in the dark. Ian was keen to go. "It sounded a fun thing; a break from the usual routine, flying to Munich and then taking the train across Germany to Hamburg. It was a big adventure; 'Ian and Jonathan go large.'"

Jonathan had seen Ian in hospital, in their homes, and in various pubs and cafes— all safe places. New places were an adventure, but they would also put Ian under pressure as he navigated through unfamiliar airports, stations, and labs. Asking Ian about the trip 20 years later, Jonathan anticipated him reminiscing about the places and people. His memories, however, were very different:

I had flown to Jersey a couple of times since my illness, but not abroad. Airports are big and unpredictable. There are so many questions. How far from the terminal to the plane? Are there stairs or an air bridge to the plane? Standing in queues was a problem. I hate them because they move too slowly. Just balancing upright and then the start/stop, with people milling around, can be disastrous. Walking is relatively easy; once I get a rhythm going I can keep going, but just standing still is probably one of the most difficult things to do.[1] To do this and chat to someone is really difficult.

Escalators are a no-go area; getting on and off scares me. I have no control over the moving walkways and am not able to think quickly enough.[2] I have never put a foot onto a moving platform; it's too risky. If I got on to an escalator I could not think enough to balance, and there is nowhere to fix my eyes on.[3]

Stairs are not a big problem; even when wide I can use one hand rail. The problem in an airport is the people rushing around. I would get someone to walk behind me to protect my back and make sure no one can run into me. Going up stairs is easier than going down, since managing weight is easier. It really throws me if steps are different heights. I like the rhythm of stairs. But at the end they often have a shallower step; that's when most falls happen. And the hand rails usually end before the end of the stairs, whereas they should end sometime after. I always check the whole stair before I get on. Always.[4]

I prefer lifts, but I do get panicked in them because of claustrophobia.[5] If it is a very small or busy lift, when I may not see my feet, then I stand leaning against a wall.

I always grab a hand rail for safety. People jostling are not good; I keep people away if I can. I always look for the panic button and stay near it, and don't like to go into a lift alone.

Travelling with Ian in unfamiliar places revealed his vulnerability and strategies far more than seeing him in his usual haunts. Around his house, the hospital, and in various cafés he was comfortable and in control. At Heathrow, in contrast, he was having to predict and calculate the whole time on the fly; how far, how many steps, how many people might be around, where was safe, where could he rest? Linda once observed that Ian's eyes were never still when he moved, as he predicted, calculated, and controlled his walking while avoiding obstacles and threats.[6] This was far more evident in these unfamiliar spaces. After the departure lounge came the next challenge.

"Getting into a plane is always exciting; is it an air bridge or steps?" Steps up to a plane from the tarmac are usually not only flimsy and steep, but they also move with passengers' weight. Neither are Ian's favorite. "I prepare and wait till the end of boarding. I don't stand in a queue and shuffle forward. If it is an air bridge ramp I'll see how steep and long it is. Are there hand rails? What is the lighting like? Is the surface slippery? How many other people are there?" Boarding was not the end of it:

> The worst bit was getting to the seat on the plane, with the narrow gangway, having to squeeze into a seat or go across the seats with no easy hand moves. The worst seats for me are those in the middle, with people either side. At London and Munich we had an air bridge. But there were a lot of steps between the air bridge and the arrival lounge. Once in Germany I went for a pee. I can't use inflight toilets because the environment of an aircraft in flight is too unstable for me.

Even now, more than two decades later, Ian's memories of going to Germany are of the moves he made and the obstacles faced:

> For a short time I would remember all the distances and the stairs, though not the number of steps [after all, once he has a rhythm this part is less demanding]. I could walk you through hotels I have not been to for years; where the lifts are and the restaurant and how far one was from the other. I could tell you about a couple of steps up into a restaurant we used in Boston 20 years ago. It is my life, how I manage. I need to find ways of being safe and finding short cuts where possible. I have a very good memory of places, which might be different to yours.

Before that plane journey Ian had never sat in a seat where he could not see his toes and where he could not stand up by putting his nose over his toes and pushing up. The plane seat in front was only inches from his nose and, as we arrived, he had to work out how to get out of the seat. It took him 10 minutes to devise a way to get up without putting his back out. In Odstock he had learned to stand from a chair by positioning his chin over his feet and pushing up. If his head was too far forward then the push would propel him forward and he would fall; if too far back then he would fall backwards; the first act of standing is positioning his head.

Ian went to Germany for experiments with Horst Mittelstaedt, a professor at the Max Planck Institute at Seeweisen, just outside Munich. He had arranged to meet Ian and Jonathan at the airport.

In the arrival hall, as the crowd thinned, they saw a man with a long leather coat and a black beret; that had to be him. They imagined he was looking for them, but he never approached, even when the place was nearly empty. So, in the end, Jonathan went up to him. As they went to the car Horst explained that he had just given his other car to his wife because it was too slow. That was an Audi Quattro; no slouch at the time. He had replaced it with a Lancia Integrale turbo, essentially a semi-tamed rally car. Ian remembers it well:

> It was quite a boys' toy. We set off down the autobahn at 200 km plus; he drove enthusiastically while chatting away. Even for neuroscientists, Horst was a lunatic driver.[7] You might remember the experiments and I remember the journey but we both remember the car ride; a shared experience of sheer horror.

Then, suddenly, they left the autobahn and were zooming down pitch-black lanes. Horst was going so fast that they overshot his institute. One U-turn later he screeched to a halt outside the lab, but was unable to find the way in through the massive gate. He disappeared to find help and Ian and Jonathan were left for 5 minutes or more, in the pitch dark, with a December mist seeping in. "Being in the car was not a problem, sitting with a seat belt round me; the dark was." Horst reappeared. He had never tried to get in so late before and had overshot the card sensor to open the gate. Once inside they were shown their residential block.

> Out the car and straight out onto a black smooth surface, through a door and immediately we were in an inner lobby, creamy light marble effect stairs with black facing. Two hand rails and then on the first floor turn right and right again and your door was on the right and mine on the left. The room was like a student's, flat level, single bed, easy access, bathroom and window overlooking a courtyard. Had the stairs been difficult I am not sure what I would have done.

The Max Planck Institute for Behavioral Physiology was set up in 1954 to study bird behavior in a natural setting. The Institute was a modest collection of labs and buildings, all sitting around a small lake. This was Lorenz's lake, where he had studied goose ethology, work for which he had been jointly awarded the 1973 Nobel

Prize, with Karl von Frisch and Nikolaas Tinbergen. Mittelstaedt was appointed in 1960 to study whole-body orientation. Ian was thrilled by its history:

> I knew about Lorenz's work but unfortunately only got to see the lake from a balcony upstairs. Being where the imprinting between geese and humans was explored and documented, wow . . . I was beside myself with joy. At one point I went into one of the rooms on campus and a sparrow-hawk was just sitting there, on a balcony rail 8 feet away from me. Horst told me that they were regular visitors, which surprised me. I'd have thought their presence would have buggered up the geese research.

Mittelstaedt's research focused on how organisms orientate their bodies in space. His particular interest in Ian's condition was in the whole-body Z-axis, which goes horizontally front to back in the sagittal plane, as opposed to the X- and Y-axes, which are left to right through the body (transverse plane) and vertically head to toe from front to back (sagittal plane) respectively. To find out how Ian orientated his whole body in space, Horst had planned two experiments which, of necessity, were in the dark on moving platforms.

In the first Ian lay on his side on a table which tilted up at the foot end, and was positioned with his inner ears at the fulcrum of movement, so his vestibular apparatus in the inner ears would provide no clues. He was strapped in safely and then, in the dark, the bottom of the table rose up slowly. His task was to return the table, still in the dark, to where he felt horizontal to be by means of a motor controlled by a bite bar between his teeth. Ian was hazy about how he did the experiment. "Laying on my side, strapped to a bed, was not so much a problem, but when the lights went out and they moved me, I was not sure where I was, nor what was happening."

They had decided on a bite bar because he could not hold anything in his hands reliably in the dark. On the last test, the tilt table stuck. They put the lights on immediately to rescue him.

> Anxious about where I was, in the dark, it was pretty scary. I am unsure how I moved back. Laying on my side on the bed, in my mind I would freeze that position. Then, with no instruction to move, I know that anything I felt was being imposed on me. I heard the machine move the tilt table and my leg felt slightly colder and more uncomfortable and there was some tension on my shoulder. I pressed the bite bar and then waited till I felt comfortable again as in the position I started. I did not know if I was right or not.
>
> I remember the tilt table broke and the lights being switched on and having to be rescued. I found myself at an acute angle with my head inclined towards the ground and my feet in the air. Oh joy. I suddenly became very interested in the integrity of the straps and the fastenings. Fortunately, Horst and his team had collected enough data, and the guinea pig survived. So much for German engineering, it didn't bode well, I was—to say the least—a little unsettled.

Over the years he can remember how he got to a lab and how he got around in it far more than the experiment itself. He does not remember the tests themselves, or the strategy he used to undertake them. He sees his responsibility as presenting himself ready and prepared for the experiment:

> I remember far more about the stairs and the distance between rooms than about the experiments. I tend to forget those, they are not important to me. I always explain that I do an experiment to the best of my ability and am happy to explain how I do it at the time. But after that it is not something which is part of my life; it is like a game, a challenge to myself. But once it is over it is over.

This can lead to difficulties in experiments. Though he might walk through a lab using the same steps each day, he might use one strategy to move during the experiment one day and another, with different results, the next. Other deafferented participants are the same, and experiments have to be designed carefully to take this into account. It is always essential to ask precisely how Ian does a given task, each time.

Fortunately, by the time the table motor broke Horst had sufficient results. After a break, Ian was shown into a windowless high-ceilinged lab the size of a gym. Horst explained that he had built it when he was appointed a professor and, to make sure it was aligned exactly north–south, he had taken his own bearings from the North Star. At one end was a large apparatus made from metal struts and small girders, open on all sides, with a large turntable contraption and a horizontal metal sled, 10 feet up. It looked like a human turntable, and that was exactly what it was.

> I don't remember being told I would be hoisted 10 feet in the air, strapped to a sled, and then spun round in the dark. Following the earlier debacle I was massively apprehensive. It was, remember, our first trip away and a learning curve for us all, and what a steep curve it had become. In fairness Jonathan was as surprised as I was. This was a monster contraption clearly dreamt up by someone with access to a scrap yard and too much time on their hands. Willie, Horst's small but agile assistant, swung around the contraption like a gibbon in tree tops. I wanted to go home.

Gamely, Ian asked if it was safe. "Yes," said Horst, "it was passed last week by the German Fairground Federation." Ian tried to look reassured. Later he said, "Remember, Mittelstaedt is a neuroscientist, and you know what they are like."

Ian was strapped into a small bucket seat and hoisted up. He shuffled onto scaffold beams with loose planks and then onto the sled where he lay on his side and was strapped down and given the (mended) bite bar. The sled was to spin round (horizontally), with Ian's ear in the center of the rotation. Once at a certain speed the sled would go out horizontally and Ian had to use the bite bar to move the sled inwards again until he felt he was back to the start position, all in the dark. The bench had measured the Z-axis when still; the aim now was to measure it when Ian was spinning since Horst thought these perceptions relied on different sensory nerves. Normally when spun outwards we feel as though we are being lifted higher at our feet, even though we are not.

After several runs, just as in the morning, there was a problem. The bite bar did not work, so Ian spat it out and shouted. Willie switched the motor off and as the turntable slowed down, he also put the lights on, allowing Ian vision as well as vestibular sensations of spin and deceleration. "As soon as I could see, I felt sick. Laying on my side being spun, and slowing down with the lights on, I felt ill, really ill, though fortunately I was not sick; just water brash on the mouth." It took him a while to recover, and to work out a plan to get down. This was a key event in his fledgling "career" as a guinea pig and a lot was learned. The science was undoubtedly good, but risk had to be minimized.

The experiments showed that Ian had normal perception of the Z-axis when spinning round (the dynamic condition), but that his judgment lying on the table was no better than expected by chance. Dynamic perception appears to depend on small sensory nerves from the gut which project through the long cranial vagus nerves (which are intact in Ian), but static perception requires large sensory nerves from the kidney capsule which had been affected by the neuronopathy. In the dynamic condition Ian behaved like subjects who have had their kidneys removed or who have complete spinal cord injuries at the neck.[8]

That evening Horst kindly asked them for dinner at his house. Jonathan remembers a pleasant evening with Horst and his wife. Ian remembers rather more:

> Inside there was a long sweeping, curving staircase with one hand rail. We discussed the war. He was an expert on the Battle of Jutland and re-created it with pretzels; as each boat sunk he ate it. He was charming. We talked a lot, but I remember the stairs and the battle.

Next day Horst took Ian and Jonathan for a drive into the foothills of the Alps, covered by then with the first snow. Horst stopped the car at the side of the road to let them see a church. They got out and he went off to park the car. Ian realized immediately that they were surrounded by ice and he was marooned; so when Horst came back they asked him to collect the car and they drove off again straight away. Ian could not understand how Horst could know his problems in the lab but then overlook them, the following day, in the real world.

Next day they were due in Hamburg, several hundred miles to the north. Planning the trip, the night sleeper had sounded exciting, but the reality was less so:

> Trains are awkward for me. With old fashioned ones the big steps up and down are very difficult, continental trains especially so. Fortunately the train was starting from this station, so I had time to plan what to grab onto, how high each step was, etc. We shared a compartment with two bunks. I gravitated to the bottom one.

It was still pitch black when, around 5 a.m., they were woken by a man with a bread roll and coffee; cold countryside slipping by as the day dawned. Two hours later they were met in Hamburg by Rolf-Detlef Treede who ferried them to his lab in a VW camper van. Ian remembers how difficult the seats were. After more rolls and coffee, work began.

The lab had one recording room well screened off from the other areas where a laser was used to heat small areas of skin very rapidly and transiently, allowing analysis of brain signals as a result of a pure heat signal to the skin. These were known to travel along small myelinated nerves termed A-delta fibers. Jonathan had previously used high-intensity electrical stimuli to show that activation of these fibers led to cortical electrical potentials recorded from Ian's scalp. Rolf-Detlef wanted to show, as a start, that Ian had similar evoked potentials from A-delta heat fibers.

The machine was mounted on a slab of granite from a local monumental mason; the laser was so powerful it could cut through metal, Bond style. Rolf-Detlef was quite proud that it was one of the few tombstones bought with a research grant. To avoid sensitizing the skin the laser was moved to a different spot on the back of the hand or foot each time, and the responses from Ian's brain were recorded through electrodes placed on his scalp. He had to wear dark glasses because of the intense laser-emitted light. The experiments proceeded very slowly, since after each stimulus to the hand or foot the laser had to be moved by a goggled assistant. The experiments required nothing of Ian except for him to stay still and keep awake. After a sleepless night on the train Ian was tired. The experiments took all day and then, around 5 p.m., they asked if he minded doing another short one. It was difficult to say no.

These were two experiments, the first stimulating receptors directly after paring some top skin away. This did not seem to work and so they stopped:

> I knew the test was not going well but didn't have the confidence to say so. Eventually Jonathan stepped in and, much to my relief, stopped it. I have a much more confidence now, and while willing to experience some discomfort, I would step in if I felt

the need. It's a difficult balance between researcher and subject, but it should be, within reason, a collaboration.

The other was in a building away from the others in the hospital grounds. In this they sat Ian in a room which looked like a cross between a bank vault and a sauna; a wood-lined safe with a big door:

> I got in, lay down, and they lowered this huge hair dryer thing onto my head. They closed the huge door, leaving me alone inside. I was very tired and as you and the guy left the room, I asked, "How do I get out of here if you two die?"⁹ The guy said there is a push bar on the door; hit that and you get out.

It was an early machine to measure the magnetic signals associated with electrical brain waves. Once more nothing came of it. As he dropped them at their hotel, the driver said he'd be back at 9 the next day. Ian said he was tired and needed longer time. "But," the man said, "the experiments start at 9.30." Ian replied they started when he got there.

The next day, a little after 10, we started the main experiment. The hypothesis concerned a phenomenon known as secondary hyperalgesia. After a bee sting the area of skin surrounding the sting becomes sensitive so that light touch is felt more intensely and as slightly unpleasant. This sensitivity could be produced by lightly brushing the skin, say with a cloth, or by touching it with a small point such as a pencil tip (though the latter was done in experiments with von Frey filaments, short wires of different stiffness which when pressed down on the skin each gave a single known pressure). The aim of the experiment was to produce hyperalgesia in Ian and compare his perception of the brush and filament with that in control subjects, to determine whether these percepts depended on large A-beta fibers (which Ian no longer had) or smaller A-delta fibers; if the latter we expected Ian to react like control subjects, if the former then he might not feel anything.

There were two snags. Firstly, to produce a bee sting large enough for the experiment involved injecting the forearm with a large dose of capsaicin, an extract of pepper, which is very painful. Secondly, Jonathan was to go first. He summoned what nonchalance he could. Rolf-Detlef explained that the pain would last 16 minutes and he was to shout each minute about its severity, so we could calibrate Ian's pain perception with others. Ian was watching Jonathan with more than his usual attentiveness:

> I remember the capsaicin going in Jonathan's forearm and the explanations about how, when it did, it would be felt at 100% intensity which would fall off with time. When it went in he shrugged his shoulders and curled like a fetus. Nothing was

said, but the body language spoke volumes. This, I thought, is going to sting; this—undoubtedly—will hurt. We both knew it would be pain, but were surprised by the intensity. When my turn came, it did bloody hurt. I was not angry; it was just what you did for the experiment.

We had discussed it before the event and Jonathan had told me it would sting. Looking back he seems to manage these "disclosures" well giving enough information to intrigue me but not enough to scare me off.

The pain scores were preliminary to the experiment to determine whether Ian felt this halo of sensitivity around the bee sting. He did for the point or punctuate touch but not for the brush. This was interpreted as suggesting that these two sensations originate in different peripheral nerve fibers, one through the large sensory fibers Ian lacked and the other through smaller fibers which were intact. Once the experiments were over Rolf-Detlef and Jonathan left Ian with a colleague as they walked to sort out some expenses. Rolf-Detlef causally mentioned that he had already written the paper, having anticipated the results. Since some papers can take months, years, and even decades to emerge, Jonathan was surprised and impressed.[10]

When he got back to work in England people asked Ian whether they had managed to improve anything. No, he explained, he did the research to allow people to understand a little more rather than to help himself:[11]

> I don't understand the science much. I have this condition and it is unique and it allows scientists to understand other conditions better. There is an intellectual curiosity and they are trying to understand it. I would be pretty shallow if I did not assist. Mittelstaedt was a nice guy and we had a great dinner and day out with him. I would go back and do it again despite the experiments and equipment failure. Treede was precise, methodical, and slick and I felt I was just there to perform. They did not seem to want to learn as they went along. He saw me as a guinea pig.

There is a big difference between doing an experiment *on* Ian and doing one *with* him. Nearly all the work done has depended on Ian doing a movement task, so his attention and performance is crucial. Treede's experiments were largely doing something to him, when little was needed from Ian himself except to keep awake. While Ian was not enamored of Rolf-Detlef's approach, his science was excellent.[12]

Ian would do it again, but there are some things he would do slightly differently. For starters, "we'd have to look at getting on the sled." His enthusiasm for the experiments, despite the sleds and the pain, was explained in part by the excitement of travel and meeting new people, and by the chance to test himself in new ways, but these seemed insufficient. A few months later we began some research in Oxford with Chris Miall and Patrick Haggard. During this another reason for Ian's engagement with science became clearer.

Often an experiment is designed to confirm or refute a specific question, as in the previous two experiments, but sometimes more descriptive methods are used.[13] In one experiment we recorded Ian's gait and showed how he activated his calf muscles in a rhythmic way, even though he could not see them. This suggested that some residual pattern generator for walking was still present within the brain and spinal cord.[14] On other occasions we might design one experiment but then realize that the results tell us something else of more interest. This was the case in a series of experiments with Chris and Patrick in Oxford.

Patrick had a curious contraption mounted on a desk with a handle sticking out the top. Ian was asked to hold it and then the handle moved suddenly before bouncing back to where it had started. By measuring the amount of movement for a given force, it measured stiffness in the arm. Ian remembers it well. "I remember because I broke the machine. I had to grab it and resist its movement; my arm was so rigid it did not move and the motor blew up in smoke." Once the smoke had cleared Patrick mended it and tried again. It was clear that Ian held his outstretched arm so rigidly to keep it stable that they would get nowhere. So they suspended his arm from the ceiling in a small sling made from string and asked him to relax the arm a little.[15]

Normally we hold the arm outstretched in a fairly relaxed way. Ian, in contrast, found that the best way was to contract all the muscles together, front and back in the arm, creating a very stiff limb, but also one which was still:

> I do create rigid frames to be accurate. To stand I will make a good position, and make it rigid so I can hang other movements onto it. No one told me when I first stood that you needed to have two feet apart, the head slightly forward, legs rigid; no one told me that if you stuck out a left arm you had to balance the other way or you'd fall over. I learned about wide bases and being rigid, tensing all the muscles, by trial and error.[16]
>
> For the grip, I was sitting down OK, but I still had to be rigid, since when I closed my eyes I had to keep gripping it without knowing where it was in relation to me and my body. If it moved it might make me fall off the chair, so I have to have my arm and my body rigid. It wasn't the grip that was the problem, it was holding the arm in position.

In another experiment Ian sat at a table with his hand resting on the table in front of him. He was shown one of a series of objects on the table to his left. He was asked to pick up the object without seeing his arm or hand. The aim was to see whether he made a correct sized open-handed grasp for each object without visual control. The answer was yes, but the most interesting part came between trials. At the end of each grasp they asked Ian to move his hand back to the start position in front of him, still with eyes shut. He did this easily, but they had anticipated that without movement and position sense it should have been very difficult. When asked about this he was surprised at their lack of imagination, since to him it was obvious. Because he rested his hand on the table between trials, that place was warmer and he just went back to the warm place each time. Why, he wondered, did they not realize that? His use of temperature was as embedded within his world as proprioception was in theirs.

The last experiment involved Ian holding a lever in his hand, which moved backwards and forwards as he bent or straightened his wrist. The aim was to see how accurately Ian could move between small changes in positions, from one to nine between the wrist being bent or straightened, though the extremes were not near his anatomical limits of movement. He never saw his hand moving and did not know how far each movement was. How would he be able to move repeatedly between unknown positions only a small distance apart, as they asked him to move from one to five to three to seven to nine to two, etc.? Perhaps surprisingly, he was quite accurate at this. When asked for his strategy, years later, he was, understandably, a bit hazy.

"If I remember, the start point was a natural place, middle, and an easy visualization." He was reminded that he had not seen the apparatus or any of the positions he moved between. "In that case I could have visualized it and you probably trained me." Again he was reminded that he had no training. "OK. So I just had a map of my head and I did it again and again." Even without seeing it, and without any feedback of what he was doing, he had managed to move his hand back and forth between each of nine positions.[17] In particular he could find his way to the wrist being at its mid-point between flexion and extension. Patrick and Jonathan presumed he was co-contracting his wrist muscles, and so getting some feedback of effort or tension, to give him a clue about hand position. In fact, when they recorded the muscle activity in his forearm at this mid position he was completely relaxed, the opposite of what they expected. Again Ian was aware of this. "I knew that if I was not making any effort then the wrist had to be in the middle position. The wrist will always go back to the middle if I do nothing and relax. I learned that through years of experience. If you want to manage in your environment, and be safe and dexterous and not fall over and be normal—whatever that is—then you have to learn all this."

That Ian had learned the biomechanical properties of the limbs in such a way was remarkable, as was his use of temperature clues. Each of these observations had come from an experiment with another aim, and each needed Ian's own observation to explain; experiments *with* Ian not *on* him.

Patrick was a Junior Research Fellow of Christ Church, Oxford and the sweetener of the visit was to stay in college and dine at High Table. Also present was Professor PBC Matthews, a Fellow of the Royal Society, who had spent his life analyzing the muscle spindle, the sensory organ within muscles which gives information about a muscle's length and tension which underpins proprioception.[18] He was naturally fascinated to meet Ian, who lived without spindles in most of his body.

There was the kerfuffle before High Table. At the pre-meal drink in the Senior Common Room, they were worried because I was chatting to some guy who was a benefactor of the college, from some big chemical company in America. He is invited regularly and funds various projects. I could see people around hoping I was not saying the wrong thing. Actually we got on well, sharing two interests; Airedale dogs and photography. We then processed from the SCR to High Table, up a spiral stone stair case without hand rails. I had not anticipated that.

It was difficult, because usually I like a clear space in front to me, so once I get going I can keep a rhythm. Being in a procession, with someone in front of me, in a gown, I could not do that. Anyway I got to my chair and then there was grace while standing and the steward said I could not sit till after that.

Patrick remembers it well:

Dinner at High Table at Christ Church was quite a performance. Jonathan had warned me in advance that Ian would like a chair with arm rests, to ensure postural stability. The only chair with arm rests at Christ Church high table turned out to be reserved for HM The Queen, who is the official Visitor of the College. So Ian sat in the Queen's armchair, and we had a wonderful meal in the atmosphere of the dining hall, candlelight, historic pictures and all. After dinner, the High Table leaves in an organized procession via a narrow spiral staircase back down to the common room. I didn't know at the time, but this is exactly the kind of thing that challenges Ian: dark, poorly visible, precipitous, and without a hand rail. He told me the next day he didn't think he'd make it down the stairs, but apparently he took a deep breath, and just did it.

Unsurprisingly Ian also remembers the spiral stairs well. They were one challenge, and Peter Matthews another:

At the end the steward said we had to process back in a certain order, and I said, "No, I will wait till the end." Down was worse than up, in part because Peter was watching just in front, and at one point had his gown on the step I wanted to go on. I had to ask him to move. He asked how I did spiral staircases and I said I had never done one before.

Peter bombarded Ian with questions, most of which he answered, though he was typically modest. "I can talk about Airedales more easily than physiology." Peter was fascinated by Ian's movement. "Yes, he was. It is always disconcerting when you turn up at a lab and people have been kind enough to read the book and so know a lot about you and your condition. It is flattering in one way, scary in another, because they know you in a way you don't yourself."

Before Ian was exposed to some science he had few words to understand or explain his condition. "Not much was known about the condition and there just wasn't the language. That is one of the things I picked up with Jonathan and the research. Yes, it was enjoyable to have Peter interested, and he was very pleasant, but I'd rather talk about flowers and dogs."

Might the professors, whether in Oxford or Germany, have validated what he had achieved? After all, to fully understand his loss, and response to it, a degree in neuroscience comes in handy:

> You'd have to ask them. My take is this. I have got a loss and all I have ever done is got on and made the best of it. It's been a hell of a bloody journey and I would not have chosen it but I have just got on with it. There are times when I would have quite liked the interest and understanding from professors of the effort I put in. There are maybe only half a dozen who understand. It is flattering, but I am reluctant to go down that path since it might make you sound shallow. But if you break your leg and go to an orthopedic ward you could have a shared experience with a number of people and there is some comfort in that, even though each person would manage it differently. I don't have that. I cannot discuss with other people. It's like being the only child, but the only child in the world. When I try to explain to an employer, maybe because I had not slept well because I cannot switch off, it can be difficult. At least the lab people understand, which is comforting.

Ian's need to find people who understood and appreciated is one reason he was prepared to do the experiments. The only time I have heard him discuss his illness and its effects on him in detail has been with neuroscientists; only then does he know that his condition and situation is understood and appreciated fully.

FRENCH CONNECTIONS

Despite his experiences in Germany, when an invitation to Quebec arrived Ian was keen to go. Chantal Bard, the leader of the group at Laval University in Quebec, kindly met us at the airport. Like Lewis Carroll's Red Queen, she had strong views and usually expressed them. She mentioned straightaway that she was a hard taskmaster and sometimes blew hot and cold, and she was as good as her word. We had arrived with a UK film crew, led by Nick Hayward Young. He was young, long-haired, and handsome; not an ideal combination, we soon learned, to endear him to Chantal. Fortunately Michelle Fleury, Chantal's colleague, played good cop to her bad one.

The additional reason for coming to Quebec was to meet Ginette Lizotte, with whom the Laval group had been working for some years. She was a Québécois, a few years older than Ian, and had developed a similar condition at about the same age, 20. But she was more severely affected than Ian. He had lost touch and proprioception from the lower neck downwards (though the back of his head was also affected; spinal C3 level); Ginette's deficit was from the lower face down (trigeminal V3). She could not feel the lower part of her face, her lower lip, or the bottom of her mouth. She used a cigarette holder—without it she squashed the cigarette between her lips—and had to be very careful eating since she could not feel food in her mouth. She also had to think about controlling her head the whole time, since her neck proprioception had been lost. In contrast, though Ian's neck is probably at least partially deafferented (it is very difficult to test), he does not think about head control. About half the muscle spindles in the body are in the small muscles of the neck, to allow the eyes and vestibular organs to be stabilized in space, so this is a huge additional problem for her. Lastly, when she became deafferented she also had a husband and young son to look after. Without time for extensive rehabilitation, she had decided a wheelchair was the best way forward.

Ian was very concerned to avoid any competition. They would do the same experiments, but rotate so they were never in the same room at the same time. Some frisson among the scientists about how Ian had done versus Ginette was inevitable though. Looking back, Ian remembers this quite clearly:

> I am fiercely competitive by nature, but generally against myself and it's a personal thing, a way of motivating myself. But at Laval, a sports-based university, the competitive spirit was everywhere. For Chantal in particular the competitive element between Ginette and I was key, I found it distracting and inappropriate. The loser was the research.

But Ian had learned from his trip to Germany, and to various labs in the UK, and was beginning to become a more expert, less passive, subject. The group at Laval had planned a week of very carefully thought out work. But Ian and Jonathan soon realized there was a difference in approach. In experiments Jonathan had always given Ian minimal instruction on how to do a task in order see, from his first trial, how he did it and then measure how he learnt. Ian was so adept at planning and predicting that they had to capture each and every trial. Chantal's group came from a rehabilitation and sports background; its approach was to give instruction, train their subjects up, and then see how reproducibly they could do a task. Both were useful in different situations, and the present situation was Chantal's.

Peter Matthews had once challenged Jonathan—rightly—not only to observe Ian's functioning, but to experiment as well. Jonathan had presented some work on Ian's gait, which showed that during walking he activated muscles he could not see, suggesting that Ian had some residual patterns of activation he was less aware of. Yes, Peter had said, but you can do more, don't just observe—ask questions. One of the experiments in Laval was to walk Ian up and down a walkway and ask him to react as quickly as he could to a click in his ear. The hypothesis was that his reaction time would reflect his attention to the click, which in turn would reflect how much effort and attention he was giving to walking. His slowest reaction time was when he had two feet on the ground, rather than when he was mid-stride. This suggested that during the stance phase he was actively planning the next step, whereas when he was actually moving he was more in the flow and, concentrating slightly less, was able to respond to the click faster. Ian agreed:

> On the catwalk I was just concerned not to fall off, after all it was 18 inches above the floor. Your suggestion seems correct; once launched the gait step goes ahead; then it is a small management thing. There is a lot more going on when standing still; planning the next step, avoiding falling, tensing up, attending to any sway in my body. I am also usually looking around and freeze my back. It is easier to control my body weight during a movement than when just standing. It is also difficult knowing how to stop at the right point, or to get started. Controlling the dead weight or momentum of the body is a problem.[1] For that I have to predict. Lastly the runway wasn't long enough to get a rhythm going, and achieving rhythm is fundamental for smooth walking.

Jonathan did not meet Ian until 12 years after his illness. In that time Ian had done much of his own rehabilitation and learned how to walk and live independently. Jonathan was always interested to see how Ian might invent a new movement, but this was not easy. He approached any novel action in very methodical way. It would be broken down into constituents and then he would decide which of his building blocks of smaller movements he would meld together to make the new one. A good analogy is with letters of the alphabet that can be put together in different ways to make new words: Ian has certain movements, and to make a new movement he puts these together in different combinations. It is rare that he extends to a longer story without a rest, since this assembly needs a lot of effort and prediction. This analogy breaks down, however; unlike other people, who once they have learned the words/ movements don't have to think about them, Ian has to think about his, and is not entirely sure that because he had them one day, he will still have them the next.

One of Chantal's tasks, called "prediction and anticipation," seemed to offer the chance to test Ian making a novel movement. In this test the subject sits at one end of a long, flat, table-like structure, which fans out to become far wider at the other end. A series of lights is set above the far end, and these turn on and off sequentially, moving from left to right, giving the appearance of a light moving across the end of the table top. The subject holds an ice hockey puck. The idea is to aim the puck to hit the table end when the light is above it. This requires the subject to anticipate where the light will have got to by the time the puck hits. Chantal had always trained subjects up and then seen their accuracy. Jonathan's idea was to shield Ian's shoulder and arm, so he could not see it, and measure the first time he had a go. Could he create and assemble a new movement, needing to be accurate in place and forward in time, on the first occasion he tried it? He was keen to try, and though Chantal was less keen to have her protocol messed with, Jonathan insisted, and Ian was pretty good first time. He had created a movement in his mind which he had neither seen nor had feedback about, and was nearly as accurate as control subjects. Ian remembers:

> I was delighted Jonathan was firm in getting them to change their protocol to monitor the first time. It was about speed, distance, and timing. I did really well and they did not understand why. I was better than Ginette even though she had trained, which wasn't the point, and it was one of those rare times I felt like a performing monkey competing.

The task was actually more complicated for Ian, since he also had to find a way of letting go of the puck at the right time. "I knew I could not release my fingers if I gripped the puck, so I had it resting in the nub of my fingers and outstretched thumb on the table. Essentially it was then just a case of timing the push; there wasn't really any letting go as such." He also remembers the number of people milling around at the time, which he felt did not make for good science.

The Quebec group had used a mirror drawing task with Ginette some years before Ian visited. The experiment was to ask her to draw round a simple Star of David on a desk with her finger. The measurements were simply of how long it took and whether she improved each time. The trick was that subjects only had mirror-reversed feedback. Control subjects were stuck at the points of the star, and jittery as they received conflicting information about where to go. In contrast Ginette did the tracing first time, fast, without jitters, and did not improve on subsequent trials; Ginette, in fact, was better than control subjects. Their conclusions were reasonable enough, that Ginette could do mirror drawing because she did not have any mismatch between where she *saw* herself going and where she *felt* herself going through proprioception.

Jonathan was not in the room when Ian did the same test but remembers Jacques Paillard, a visiting French neuroscientist, rushing out excitedly to tell him that, "Ian got stuck." Ian's results were worse than Ginette's and close to that of controls. Ian was annoyed, though not because Ginette outperformed him:

> I was so annoyed because they made an awful lot of it. Chantal and Jacques referred to it, and how Ginette had done it without effort. Then there was a camera crew filming as well. I couldn't do it as well as I wanted and I had so much pressure. I was not happy.

It was only many years later that Jonathan followed this experiment up with Chris Miall in Birmingham. Jonathan and Chris used a more sophisticated virtual mirror and a graphics tablet which allowed them to see where subjects went, as well as how long they took to go round a series of patterns, from a simple angular loop to more complex shapes with several acute angles.

In the mirror drawing test Ian was stuck at the corners, like the control subjects. The conclusion was that Ian, like the controls, was stuck not because of a mismatch between seeing the arm moving and a feeling of where the arm is going (from proprioception), but because of a mismatch between visual feedback of where the hand is going and an internally generated motor program of where the hand is planned to go next. When doing the task, one's own introspective feeling supports this. The problem at the points of the star is felt as conflict between where one *sees* the pointer going and where one *wills* it to go, rather than between where it is seen and where it is felt (in fact one has no awareness of the latter).

This experiment was relatively simple but important since it showed that Ian uses these forward motor programs, or plans or intentions; something he has always said but which is quite difficult to show experimentally. It also revealed a crucial difference in the way Ian and Ginette move.[2] She tends to use on-line real-time visual feedback for such movements, whereas Ian makes plans for movement. Normally this allows him to move more quickly and with more complexity and control, until any visual feedback is mirror-reversed of course.

Another experiment, with Michelle, followed up some work which showed that Ginette was less able than controls to judge intervals of time, say 2 seconds to 2 minutes. These were among the most tedious experiments Ian has ever done. Locked in a room, his task was to sit there and say when he thought a period of 2 minutes had passed. This was bad enough, but then Chantal burst in to ask how things were going. Now Ian always approaches experiments with good grace and humor, but when doing the task requires all his concentration he expects others to do the same. He kept his thoughts to himself, but it was not one of the more successful experiments.

> I was with Michelle, and supposed to estimate intervals without counting . . . Half way through Chantal burst in and then left, slamming the door. I was incandescent inside, and Jonathan calmed me down as I burned off some anger pacing the corridor. Some researchers appear to have such a disregard for others' work. I vowed never to work with her again.

Jacques Paillard and Jonathan managed to smuggle an additional experiment into the schedule, a repeat of something the latter had done with Ian when first they met. How accurate could he judge a lifted weight without proprioception and touch? The underlying interest was in whether the perception of weight was all peripheral or whether it might involve a central sense of the effort. Charles Bell had wondered this when he first described awareness of position and movement in 1833:

> At one time I entertained a doubt whether this proceeded from a knowledge of the condition of the muscles or from a consciousness of the degree of effort directed to them in volition . . .[3]

The experiments were simple. Different weights were concealed in small canisters, and the task was to decide whether the next one was heavier or lighter than the last. The weights were manipulated without Ian being aware until his minimum perceived difference was found as he lifted them up. With his eyes open Ian could judge a weight as well as anyone else, around 5% liminal difference. But with his eyes shut this difference became massive, around 100%, so he could distinguish 1 kg from 2 kg, or 50 g from 100 g, but not less than that. It was suggested that with his eyes open he made a certain movement and estimated either the speed of upwards movement in his arm or its extent, and made his judgment from that. He agreed.

"I remember the little canisters, to 'guess the weight.' I used the same force each time and the same grip force and see how they reacted." It was remarkable that he could make such reproducible movements, but then he had spent years practicing.

With his eyes shut there were a number of possibilities. Jonathan had originally asked Ian to pick up the weights with his outstretched hand. Then he might have felt something different in the hand or forearm, or even at the neck where sensation was normal. He might even have judged that his head and body moved more with a larger weight, making the judgment from the inner ear.

But then Jonathan restricted Ian's movement to the forefinger going upwards with the hand resting sideways on a soft surface. Then, using only one muscle, he could still do the task, but when that muscle became fatigued the ability to judge weights was lost. Jonathan thought that this suggested strongly that Ian was using existing peripheral receptors from muscles—normally involved in the perceptions of tension and fatigue—for the crude but still impressive judgment of force. Without being able to see his movement, or feeling it as movement, a central judgment of effort seemed less likely. The same experiment was tried with Ginette one evening, with the same result. She could detect a normal weight difference (5%) between small concealed weights in boxes when she lifted then up with her eyes open but the difference rose to 100% when her eyes were shut.

Jonathan presumed she performed the task in the same way as Ian, seeing how far—or how fast—her arm moved for a given movement and weight. In a way she was a spectator to her own action. If so, then he reasoned that a group of researchers might be able to make the same judgment. Jonathan assembled a group to sit round while Ginette did the task and asked them to do the same as her, estimate the weights as being heavier or lighter than the last one by watching how she moved. Ginette now changed her strategy in a way which puzzled Jonathan. She made one fast lift initially and then a number of other lifts and falls which seemed random. Afterwards he asked her why she had made so many movements. "Well I made my judgment on the basis of my first fast movement and how the arm moved up. All the other movements I made to fool you lot."[4]

The week went quickly, with these and other experiments each done in a different room in a large underground lab. Though she blew hot and cold Chantal had arranged an excellent visit. Ian still remembers it fondly, up to a point:

> Laval was a nice place and I am pleased I went. It was a big trip for me. For the most part I enjoyed it and it was good to meet Ginette. But we needed more time together and a translator. Their research facilities were great, but I was also frustrated. They didn't seem interested in listening to another's point of view and I was disappointed to be judged against Ginette. The experiments were challenging and I enjoyed taking

part, but the competitive spirit diminished the experience, and sadly, I suspect, the research.

He had soon gone from being a relatively passive experimental subject to having his own views about the methods and quality of the science.

Not long after visiting Quebec, Ian was invited to a lab with close ties to Laval, in Marseille. All went well on the journey out, until when walking across the marble floor in Marseille airport to the car Jonathan pointed out how slippery the floor was. Ian had no idea, and stiffened visibly. It was worse outside; the mistral, a strong wind from the Alps, was blowing. So as they walked to the car Ian had to calculate how far to lean, Lowry style, into it. That was fine but just occasionally the wind slackened and he nearly fell forward.[5]

The experiments in Marseille were on the control and guidance of movements and, in particular, on the ways in which vision and arm movement were coordinated and were run by the leader of the group, Gabriel Gauthier, and his deputy, Jean-Louis Vercher. In the first Ian sat securely at a table in the dark, with his head position stabilized by clamping his teeth onto a bite bar. In front of him was a screen on which appeared two small lights, which gave no ambient light. One was in the middle of his visual field and the other moved from the center to the left around 50 degrees, either in a rapid jump or very slowly. In the complete darkness, his task was to follow the target shift in one of three ways; by a smooth pursuit of his eyes with the target, by rapid saccadic eye movement (rapid movements of the eyes that abruptly change the point of fixation) to the target once it had finished moving, or to track the movement using his peripheral vision while still fixating on the central dot. Then, he had to move his arm and hand across the table to where he thought the target dot of light had moved. It was found that he placed his arm most accurately when he had moved his eyes rapidly, in a saccade. In other words he had, unconsciously, used his central movement program to move his eyes to assist movement of his arm.[6]

This was the result; getting there proved more arduous than anticipated. Initially Ian used a sound clue, listening to his arm moving across the table to gauge how far he had gone, even without vision, by moving at a set speed and gauging the time it took. Then, at the end of each trial he was asked to return his arm to the front, and he was able to do this, despite being in the pitch black, using the same temperature clues he had mentioned in Oxford. So, to avoid temperature and noise clues, his arm and hand were wrapped in a cloth and he wore head phones playing white noise.

But he still managed to get back to the start position. It was presumed that he could do this by a process of cognition and cunning. He knew where his eyes were in his head and that the static dot was always dead in front. His head was immobilized by the bite bar and his body was also secure on the chair. So then he just had to move his arm to what he imagined, or visualized, to be the mid-point beneath him. All movement was referenced from the single small point of light he could see, an astonishing calculation in complete darkness and without feedback.

In another experiment, Jean-Louis asked Ian to watch a dot moving back and forth over a screen in front of him while his eye movements were measured. The dot moved faster and faster until it was too fast for Ian to track and, instead, he made short sharp saccadic eye movements. This was entirely normal. Next he asked Ian to control the dot's movements by moving a cursor leftwards and rightwards with his arm. Then he could track the dot during far faster eye movements than before without degenerating into catch-up saccades. In other words, he was able to quicken eye movement by coupling them with arm movement, unconsciously.[7] Jean had shown persistence of these linked motor programs, from arm to eye, even without any peripheral feedback.

Now Ian rarely goes to a lab just once. Something is usually seen that needs further study. On a second visit to Marseille, Ian's ability to move his arm back to the resting point in front of him without vision was followed up, this time doing an experiment each day, slowly and progressively stripping out any clues he might use to help him.

Ian was in a secure chair and immobilized by a bite bar, so it was certain his head could not move. This time, as before, there were two small spots of light, neither of which gave any reflected or ambient light. One was the moving target, the other was fixed in position, in the mid-point of Ian's vision. With the small target spot of light moving vertically Ian had to match his arm position by moving it up or down and then return his arm to the resting position. First Ian's performance was measured with full vision and in a lit room. Then visual clues were progressively removed. Once more, with the single spot of light in front of him, he could move the arm to track the target light and back again. But in the complete dark, with the moving target light but not the stationary reference one, he was completely lost and could neither track the moving light nor get his arm back to the start. This was one of the few times he allowed the removal of all clues. It was also potentially dangerous, since he was in complete darkness, sitting with his teeth clamped to a bite bar; if he had slipped he could have damaged his teeth or back.

His ability to move his arm under any of these conditions was an astonishing act of planning and motor imagery. Sitting in the dark with the fixed position light only, without any touch or movement and position sense, he could still move his arm with some accuracy. This was absolutely dependent on his knowing that the single spot of light in front of him was in the middle of his eyes, that his eyes were pointing ahead, that his head was rigid in the bite bar, that his body was stationary in the chair, and that his arm had limited movement. But all was absolutely dependent on one external reference point; the small spot of light. The chain of assumption about body parts and movement fell apart as soon as this was extinguished.[8]

Marseille in spring was delightful; we spent one night in Gabriel's fishing village 10 miles round the coast from Marseille and, on a day off, Jean-Louis showed us Aix-en-Provence and Avignon. But our collaborators needed time for their families and friends, and it was nice for Ian and Jonathan to relax in the evening on their own too. Le Vieux Port had a number of restaurants. Jonathan would scout one out and Ian would decide how far he could walk round to eat. In those days he was ambitious and would walk right to the opposite side of the harbor. They came back one night and had a beer in a bar.

They were sitting minding their own business when Ian said they should not be too attentive to the women at the next table who, he suggested, were working girls. Later they watched as the barman came out from behind the bar, stood behind a man chatting up some women, lit his cigarette lighter, and held it 6 inches below the man's crotch. A few seconds later the man realized that his groin was on fire. Ian and Jonathan laughed so much they thought they had better retreat. Later Ian learned from his brother, who was in the Foreign Legion stationed just outside Marseille, that this bar was off limits because it was too rough.

Ian learned fast in Canada and was no passive subject. He was concerned that the work with Ginette had colored the approach of the Laval scientists, and that they presumed Ian and Ginette were similar.

> I was a different monkey to the one they expected and they never took on board how different we are. Our strategies are different; the levels of disability different, with Ginette more affected, and our temperaments are different too. I tend to create strategies for doing tasks more than her. They assumed we were the same. We are not, and it pisses me off that researchers don't listen when you try to point these things out. It is simple, the ingredients are different, and therefore the results are different. Failure to take our differences into account must surely skew any conclusions from where we have both been guinea pigs.

He was also concerned about how involved she was during the experiments:

> For the eye and hand experiment in Marseille, we had to make the Blue Peter[9] adjustments with a sleeve on to stop me using temperature clues, and ear phones

with white noise to stop me using sound of my hand along table top. Most of the tests had already been done by Ginette. So I am thinking; did she use temperature, sound, timing like that? Why have they not stripped them out? Did she do it and not tell them? Did they not ask how she did the test? That is why I get frustrated. Firstly they compare us and then they do not seem to have asked her about how she does it. Then—even then—they make the assumption that we may use the same strategy to do a test as each other, or even as we did yesterday, neither of which are necessarily true.

Before going to Quebec, Ian had been worried that meeting Ginette would be difficult and that she might feel inadequate for not having learned to walk and stand. In fact the opposite occurred and he came away troubled himself. Seeing her living so happily and completely from a wheelchair made him re-evaluate his own motivation and effort. Why precisely had he spent so long learning to stand and walk? Why did he put himself into such precarious situations every day, when he could fall or slip at any time? Why did his expend so much energy to appear normal and upright, when he saw Ginette living so happily from a chair? Though he knew he wanted to return to normal social life and not appear different, the effort required and living with the constant risk from falling were both huge. He normally accepted them without thinking; Ginette made him question these anew.

One of the problems in Quebec was the filming. However discreet and unassuming the crew, a camera does alter the dynamic and is difficult to ignore. At times also there had been three crews, one internal to the department, one from the local TV, and another with Nick. Previously Ginette had been involved in a short TV feature for Canadian TV. Ian and Jonathan saw part of this, an interview with a local physician and neuroscientist not working with us in Laval. When he met Ginette, he told the interviewer, he had immediately realized her importance to science. "When she came in I realized we could throw the monkey out the lab." Ian, not surprisingly, was amazed:

> It was unbelievable to see this astounding statement captured on film. It confirms that there are still researchers who see you as a commodity. I am lucky I have worked with people, for the most part, who do not think like that. It shows disrespect to people and other primates.

Jonathan thought of a meeting on ethics at which Jane Goodall had spoken. When asked about research on primates she thought for a moment and then replied that she saw no reason why chimpanzees should not take part in research. As the room gasped she continued, "So long as they give their own consent."

4

HUNGRY

While in Canada Ian hinted that all was not well between him and Linda, and on his return she told him their marriage was over. Ian was devastated. There were certainly pressures on both of them. Ian needed time to relax and reflect, and then was exploring a new career in access audit with no guarantee of success. Linda was breadwinner and housewife, in a new job and a new place. Living in rented houses for several years could not have helped. Then, finding that the place they bought needed so much work, when money was tight, must have hurt them both. Their accounts differ about the causes for their breakup, as one presumes they always do.[1]

Ian left for a while, going to his mother's in Jersey for a few days. Once he was back in the Lakes Linda would not reconsider. After a few weeks of sharing the house uneasily, he came down south and stayed with friends until he found somewhere to live in Waterside, across the Solent from Southampton. It was nice enough, though not in a great area; Ian never liked it:

> It was on a bleak housing estate; all I could afford. The neighborhood was rough. I got home one day to find the road blocked off. The man opposite was being threatened by his son with a gun for sleeping with his girlfriend. The police were often going up and down doing drug raids. I affectionately nicknamed it Beirut, though my neighbors were absolutely fabulous and exceedingly helpful.

It was a grim time. Alone, unemployed, and broke, he could hardly afford a bar of chocolate. His small work pension and benefits were pitifully insufficient, and he wasn't prepared to "milk the system" like so many around him. He had worked so hard to become mobile. Now, after two marriages and a decade in work, he felt back to square one:

> All those dreams, hopes, and aspirations had amounted to nothing. The onset of my disability and rebuilding myself had been a struggle, but this was devastating. I remember seeing an old acquaintance I knew through Linda at a petrol station; she scurried off to avoid speaking. It was hard to pick yourself up.
> After a while I found myself again and started to build my future; I'd show them, all of them, and I would do it for me. On one level I knew I had the resilience and

character to cope, my disability had given me that. But I had never been so scared or frightened in my life. If only I had known what adventures and fun were ahead.

Ian did not want to return to his old job in the Civil Service; apart from the tedium he would be going back having lost his wife and his independence; it would have been like returning to Colditz. He had enjoyed the Holiday Care Service work, and continued to work for them, but they only paid expenses. He needed more. One hope was that the Disability Discrimination Act (DDA) was coming out in a few years' time, and he knew that would generate work in access audit.

He found a company in the Yellow Pages, Disability Matters, that was doing access audit work locally, rang them, and arranged to meet the boss, Stephen Duckworth:[2]

> He was inspiring and amazing. He broke his neck playing rugby and is tetraplegic. He continued to study, qualified as a doctor, and then went into disability studies. He had his own company advising other companies how to become accessible. One of his other niches was getting disabled people back into employment. I thought if he could do all this, and have a family, from a wheelchair, then I must be able to make a go of it.

Stephen suggested a self-improvement course designed to assist people return to work, "as a springboard." It was a 6-week course spread over 3 months, and combined practical advice with workshops on increasing self-esteem. Stephen had found that people who are unemployed due to disability are hampered as much by their loss of self-confidence as by their impairment. He chose good hotels, with excellent coffee[3] and proper lunches, to show his clients they did not always have to make do with the cheap option. Living alone, the lunches were especially welcome to Ian.

Ian impressed; 2 weeks into the course they offered him a job with the company. Ian bit Stephen's hand off and at the end of the course started as a freelance consultant. "I knew I was as good as anyone else working for Holiday Care Service. I thought I could do it. Stephen and Mike Freeney, his assistant, said, 'Join us for a few weeks and see how it goes.'" After 6 weeks Stephen said that they reckoned that if they didn't take Ian on he would be their competition in a few years, which was really encouraging. "They knew I was hungry. I wanted to work, not live off the state; I wanted to earn a living, doing something I enjoyed. I wanted to compete on a level playing field with the rest of them."

Stephen was very supportive, though he was so busy he had little chance to teach Ian. In fact they only went to one presentation together, in Cambridge:

> His PA drove while Steve read papers; he was never one for chit chat. He did an amazing presentation and then asked me to stand up and write on the board. I can write, and I can stand, but I had never done the two together, so I said no and his PA did it.

On the way out I told him why I could not do it. He was very good; it was no problem and he just accepted it. I thought that was cool. In the Civil Service a manager once asked me to attend a meeting and take minutes. I had done this before, but did not think this manager would help me if I needed it, and I also knew he was fastidiously picky, so I said no. He said, "Fair enough. I will never recommend you for promotion," and he was true to his word.

One of Ian's first trips was with Mike to the Cinema Exhibitors Association in London. They were worried about how the DDA would affect the cinema industry since most of the UK's cinemas at that time were old and inaccessible. "Mike arranged to meet at the train station. I had not done trains, so it was very scary. It was an early start from Salisbury, nowhere near where I lived, so I had to get up very early indeed." There was a long walk from the booking office to the platform, down a long ramp under the tracks and up again. There were hand rails, though he had to rest three or four times going down and up. Just getting to the platform was a journey.

Fortunately the train started from Salisbury so there was time to get on, but at the London terminal he had to get off. "Getting off, managing my weight coming down was more difficult than getting on. I managed it, though by now Mike had legged it to get a taxi." Mike knew little about Ian's problem. Ian had tried to explain once but ended up suggesting he had a bad back, which seemed easier all round.[4] Ian got to the taxi rank and stood in the queue trying to impress Mike:[5]

> We got to the meeting and went upstairs. The boss, John Wilkinson, was loud, a smoker, thought rude by 90% of those he met and the most politically incorrect person I have ever met. He was old school and old tie, but I loved the guy. John was the most influential and effective person I ever met in the cinema industry. Together with industry stalwarts like Barry Keward and Tom Allinson from Odeon, he changed accessibility within cinemas throughout the UK. No more being wheeled in through a fire door to be parked at the front, with the wheelchair user destroying their neck as they cradle upwards to see the silver screen. Most cinemas in the UK were built before the war and access was never a consideration. Effecting change was going to be tough and if I was part of the team I knew it was going to be one hell of a ride.

After a while Mike suggested they audit some cinemas. Ian was not backward in pointing out the absence of hand rails or that there were too many steps. One auditorium was down two flights of stairs. Ian showed them in person how awkward it was for him, let alone for someone in a wheelchair:

> I was very vocal and told them what it was like for me. What I needed would be good for others; easy access was good for everyone. If I could not read the signs in a quick glance the others could not either. In one cinema the patterns on the carpet were quite confusing so anyone with a visual impairment might miss a step. Apparently

someone had fallen there a few weeks earlier and was suing. It was all basic stuff, but they listened.

Back at their office Mike asked Ian for his opinion the whole time. Mike, it turned out, understood the DDA well enough but was weak on the physical access side. The Odeon's management was obviously very pleased with the day, since they asked the company to audit their cinemas and, moreover, asked Ian to do it. That day he went from being nobody to someone who charged £300 a day. Over the next months and years he audited over 100 cinemas. He reckons he has seen 60–70% of the cinemas in the UK, cutting his disability access audit teeth as he went.

Before Ian no one had thought of a detailed access audit template to use across buildings. He developed one to give continuity across the cinema industry and used it initially for all Odeons and then for all the other cinema operators. In the process Disability Matters found itself one of the leading companies in the UK for disability access and Ian was one of their main consultants. The next few years were busy, lucrative, and exhausting; he audited most of the familiar banks and building societies on the high street, major retail chains, hotel chains, Regional Health Authorities, and the Post Office:

> A bank is actually very similar to a hospital. In a hospital it is access to the car park and then from there to the outpatient appointment or ward. With both it is access into the building and then in a hospital it is massively about signage and understanding the shortest, levelest route. People have tried lots of ways for signage. You just can't have signs to all the places at all places; that is too much information. At the reception in the Royal Free Hospital in London there was a massive board with directions to a hundred departments. A woman sat underneath there to tell you where to go; no one could read the bloody sign.

When Ian audited Odstock Hospital, where he had been a patient, he found color-coded floors, but they were too pastel and even people working there were lost. He mentioned this at a meeting in Marlborough where they were designing a new hospital. A man at the front blanched; he had been responsible for Odstock. Generously, he agreed they had learned lessons.

> Color use can't be subtle and should be combined with shape; say a red ladybird and a green frog in a children's hospital. You'd think a hospital would be sympathetic to disabled people, but absolutely not. A hospital is a machine with operates effectively and efficiently for its staff but not necessarily for the patients who come in to feed it. Banks are relatively easy, though much of the portfolio is old, with listed buildings, musty old things. They are a nightmare for access. Even though the Act says you need level access, try doing that in a Lutyens' doorway.

One client was the large retail chain John Lewis. He and Mavis used to go there for a treat. At that time he thought them upmarket and snobbish. Now he was a consultant for them:[6]

> I remember having a cup of coffee in their Kingston store thinking it surreal; 5 years before I would never have dreamt of doing this. I got flashbacks about my journey, remembering how far I had travelled. Mavis would have been delighted.

Auditing Adtrans, a company in Derbyshire making trains and carriages, the boss told Ian to be careful around the site, but otherwise to go wherever he wanted. By this time he had begun to use a wheelchair for difficult sites and for this one he took Dave Hopkins, a friend, as an enabler. The buildings were massive, with carriages coming in one end broken and going out the other shiny and mended. You would turn a corner to find a train coming towards you. He went into one shed, larger than a football pitch, when someone jumped out the office and asked if he was doing the disabled access. Since Ian was being pushed by Dave this was a good guess. He wanted Ian to look at a carriage with an accessible toilet being installed for a UK rail firm:

> I got out the chair, up into the carriage and he showed me the toilet. I said it doesn't work. People in a wheelchair would not be able to transfer to use it, especially going along a track at 70 miles per hour. I talked him through it and justified my comments. We shook hands and off I go.

Later that week Ian was in the same shed when another man approached. He was the head designer and wanted to go through the issues. There was a group of people in the carriages so Ian asked if they should wait. He insisted, so Ian got up into the carriage and went through the toilet problems all over again. The man was clearly disappointed but could see Ian's point. As he went to leave, two people from the other party in the carriage approached him and asked him to go over the points once more. They were from the train company buying the carriages and had come to sign off the final contract. After hearing Ian's opinion they refused to do it:

> I got off the train and apologized to the guy who had asked me to get on in the first place. He said that obviously the Chiltern Trains man was very angry, but that it was not my fault since he had asked me to go on. I looked around for Dave to continue with the main audit, the reason that we had been in the shed in the first place. But he had disappeared. Some moments later he returned and whispered to me through the side of his mouth, "I have been to get the car and it's parked outside, just in case we need to make a quick getaway."

The contract Ian had just derailed was for around £10 million. He phoned his office to find out how much the company was insured for. About £10 million they said. Ian thought he'd just spent it. The Adtrans' boss asked to see him within minutes. Ian apologized. To his credit the boss said it was not Ian's fault. In the end they redesigned the toilets and the carriages went out. "It was a bit of a cheek. I never did get a consultancy fee for the advice I gave. But I did learn a valuable lesson; to be sure, always use the toilet before you get on a train."

The episodes highlighted that accessibility should be part of the design during development; fortunately this inclusive design is now happening far more. Ian has worked in this way with John Lewis and several hotel groups:

> People often think of me as the spawn of Satan with unreasonable expectations for access provision and for costing them money. But it just isn't the case. Given the opportunity to initiate an "inclusive design" concept we can, and do, save our clients money.

One day he had a phone call asking him to audit The Dorchester. As one of the top hotels in London he was very interested. He got to Park Lane at 9 a.m. prompt:

> It is so different from other hotels. We arrived in a taxi to be met by a doorman who got the wheelchair. I dropped my pen and before I could reach down there were two people picking it up. The service was amazing. But—unbelievably—I couldn't get in through the front door so entered through a side door which led into a kitchen. When the manager arrived we showed him the appalling access for disabled guests. He replied that Christopher Reeve had used the same entrance without complaining.

Ian was not impressed and replied "Maybe, but I don't fly." "I was astounded" says Ian, "The Dorchester had such low expectations for their guests with disabilities, even though you can guarantee that they charged them the same rates." In one of the suites overlooking Hyde Park he suggested widening an internal door, adding that the cost might be high. The facilities manager said, "There is no such thing as 'No' at the Dorchester; if that is what the guest wants that's what the guest gets." Well, Ian thought, except for access through the main entrance to the hotel for those with a disability.

Ian eventually reached the ground floor toilets. The ladies smelled lovely and had style, the gents smelt of sandalwood and was equally posh. In contrast, the accessible toilet was bog standard. All it told Ian was that they considered disabled people second-class citizens. The facilities manager was not pleased to have this pointed out, but needed to be shown that disabled people should be treated like everyone else.

Ian has been in a lot of ladies' toilets. Once, in a small museum in Dorchester, he had to audit the ladies, so he asked an elderly lady to go in to make sure it was free and then had her standing outside stopping people go in:

> I was explaining that you need to make it the right color and well lit for people with visual impairments. She said you'd soon know if you were in the gents "it smells because the men all pee on the floor." The ladies', in contrast, she said, "really did smell of lavender."

In a few years Ian had gone from nowhere to heading a successful business. One of his mantras had been to turn misfortune to his advantage. While his impairment undoubtedly led him to access audit, it also deepened the way in which he saw space and people's movement through it. He had several years of punishingly hard work, but work the pace and amount of which he could control. Sometimes he would be away for 10 days, in a different bed each night, doing two or three audits per day; hard work even without his impairment. But, even at its most hectic, it was better than the dreaded 9 to 5 office job. He earned good money and he controlled what he did.

He also realized that though his parting from Linda was intensely painful, he would never have done all this if he had stayed with her.[7] He had picked himself up once more through hard work and sheer personality and could now afford all the chocolate he wanted. Next on the list was moving house.

L'HOMME QUI

Jonathan picked up the phone one evening and a voice asked if he had heard of Peter Brook. It was Marie-Hélène Estienne, Brook's collaborator and dramaturge, phoning from Paris. They were working on a new play adapted from Oliver Sacks' book, *The Man Who Mistook His Wife for a Hat*. They had heard, she explained, of Ian and his disability; might he go to Paris to assist Peter and his company develop their portrayal based on Oliver's essay on Christina, "The Disembodied Lady"? Jonathan phoned Ian; he was not familiar with Brook, but had heard of Paris and was up for the trip.

Brook's theater, Bouffes du Nord, was built in the late nineteenth century with two balconies; the performance space is set in the round on the ground floor. Behind this, under and beyond the proscenium, where there might have been a stage, the space extends backwards on the same level. The huge wings and back of the space are bare in a deep, beautiful terracotta color. Brook's company was even more exotic. Sotigui Kouraté was a tall, lean figure from Mali, Yoishi Oida was more heavily built and Japanese, Bruce Myers was an English actor, while the musician, Mahmoud Tabrizi-Zadeh, was from Iran; they all moved with the silence of stalking panthers. Ian was to be portrayed by David Bennent, a Swiss, who had been with Brook for several years, having been a child actor in *The Tin Drum*. All were very welcoming and had a presence which Ian and Jonathan felt. The company, the space, and Brook's welcome were intoxicating; this was to be an adventure.

David and Ian went out for a meal that evening and the next day Peter allowed Ian to take part in his warm-up exercise for the actors. Then they went through how Ian stood and how he moved. Peter drew out of Ian the fine detail, looking at him in a different way from the scientists. Rather than experiments and apparatus, Peter's tools were his gaze and his questions. He explained that they had been research-ing the play for over 6 months and had initially found it very difficult. An actor, he explained, would explore a character from "the inside out," trying to look and feel his own emotions and expand them in relation to those of his character. If the play was about, say, jealousy, then the actor would look inside to his own experience and seek to use that to begin his characterization, amplifying it to Shakespearean levels if necessary. They had been fascinated by Oliver Sacks' stories of people with neurological and neuropsychological impairments, and had started by trying to portray them in workshops. But with no experience of their own that they could use to flesh out Sacks' case studies, they got nowhere. Their solution was to go back, beyond Sacks' accounts, to find similar patients in Paris and elsewhere. By seeing these subjects as people, not just as cases, they could begin to understand them. In an interview about the process Bennent described it thus:

> It was absolutely the contrary of The Tempest, where we already had the power . . . from Shakespeare's existing play. For The Man Who there was nothing. Our concrete start- ing point in rehearsal was a 4-month rehearsal period in hospitals in Paris, studying particular illnesses and case histories. Our task was to observe and act exactly in accordance with the specific forms of the illness in minute detail. We went into the hospitals every day; in the evenings we talked and started to write. In this way we gradually built the piece and then we rehearsed it for a further 3 months.
>
> At first we could not understand what was going on inside, so we had to take the ex- ternal movements and behaviors of these patients and just work on the outside forms of these personalities, which is why it was sometimes very difficult for us. We could 'do' a movement, having watched it from the outside, but we couldn't understand it, especially, for me, with the character who has lost proprioception of his own body. Peter had found a book by the neurologist Jonathan Cole about this patient; we had read it, had been moved by the story, and wanted to include it; not everything came from Oliver Sacks, that was just a base. At the time I said to Peter, I am completely lost, I have read about this man I know a little about him, I know how he moves, but I don't understand him. And I am absolutely incapable of playing him because when I do it is exclusively external.
>
> So Brook asked if the patient could come over with his doctor to Paris and he came for 1 week and it was extraordinary. Then I could watch him, and see his external movements, but he could explain to me in detail and speak to me about his sensations and feelings. This was a great help, because from then on I could begin to go a little further inside.[1]

Ian had no previous experience of theater or of acting:

> I had not heard of Peter Brook. But the thought of going to Paris, and meeting him was too good an opportunity. When we met I was awe-inspired. He has such a presence. I am not au fait with the theater and may not have given him due deference. He sat there patiently and generously and said the theater is about engaging, enthusing and engaging, and not just about the story. It was how he managed his group which was inspiring. He was so revered in his arena and yet he was very generous in how he moved forward, as a community thing. It was not that he wrote it and told the others, he moved forward as a group.
>
> It took a second or two to get my head round that he was portraying me. I was quite happy with it. I thought it was good stuff; in fact I was bowled over. A butcher from Jersey sitting in the theater with one of the world's leading directors asking how to

portray me. That is what it made it comfortable; I was able to talk about something they did not know so well. I was immediately put at ease talking about how I managed to walk, to stand, or to hold a cup.

Though at ease, it was still an ordeal. The whole company observed Ian in minute detail. Ian had been in this situation before, though in labs rather than the theater:

> I find it humbling, and I can feel guilty in labs, where people have read the book and papers, since they ask questions about me and I cannot always remember. In Paris they did try to pick me apart. They got part of me but not others, and certainly not my humor. It is unnerving when you know that from the second you set foot in the theater you are under a microscope and you know the actors are following every detail, and that every mannerism might be portrayed back and then you have to critique what they did.

Peter was interested in Ian's movement and pose; his "performance." This led Ian to question whether Peter saw him for what he was, "just a guy performing his way through life?" Unlike the neuroscientists, Peter was less interested in the technical side of Ian's movement but rather how he looked. Ian was disconcerted since Peter touched on something that he usually skirts around:

> He stripped me down to "images" of how I looked at various stages, in standing, walking, and sitting. All this was getting close to the real me, not just the movement but the "façade," and how or why I chose to portray myself in certain ways. I rarely touch on why I put so much effort into "performing," because I don't want to be perceived as artificial or false. I have really struggled with this issue over the years, but it is something I manage better now. We all have an image of ourselves, and the way we want the world to see us. I just have to take it a touch further to stay safe and avoid falling over.

During the course of the week David and Peter evolved a way of representing Ian and his condition which was truthful and which allowed them to communicate with an audience, even if, for Ian, it was not exactly him. For his part Jonathan saw times when David was clearly doing something that Ian would not—could not—do. He stood up, for instance, snapping his knees to brace them with a jerk. Ian did not notice that, but when Jonathan pointed it out he did not mind.

> Jonathan was better at observing it from the outside. I looked at it from the inside. They wanted to show me standing and I showed them how I did it. But they could not let go of the proprioception I don't have. Even though they tried to try to take it away, in portraying me, you just cannot switch it off.

In a way this did not matter. While, of course, it is not possible to move as though without proprioception, one can show something of the constraints with which Ian lives. David's portrayal had a deep sincerity; a realistic, sympathetic representation which allowed others to understand the condition, and then identify with the person living with and exploring it.[2] It was the only vignette in the play taken from a single person's experience rather than from a number of subjects with the same condition. Because of this, however, it had to have its own life, faithful to Ian's experience but not slavishly aping it. How extraordinary to help someone act you, trying to capture your condition but also something of you, yourself.

In the play David, lying on two chairs, as in bed, under a sheet, began by explaining his condition and situation:

PATIENT. "I've lost all sensation of my body. My head moves, but from my neck to my feet I can't feel my body any more. If I don't look at it, I don't know it's there, it's as if it does not exist. The doctors explained to me that I'm not paralyzed. They say I've lost my proprioception."

He then spoke the poem Ian had written while in Salisbury Hospital at the beginning. Its power on the page was heightened by being portrayed live:

Living Death

Turned every two hours
Like a joint of meat.
Unmoving like a statue,
Mind filled with emotion.
Limbs dead to the touch,
Movement impossible.
Lying on a bed eyes fixed
On a flaking ceiling.
Wishing those flakes
Would turn to cracks,
And the ceiling fall, to
Take me from this misery.
What use an active brain
Without mobility.

Stage Direction. The Patient now moves slightly and discovers his body.

"I've found out that if I look at my arm I can guide with my eyes. Only my eyes can help me. I must use them to direct my hand towards the sheet, I take hold of it by closing my fingers, I can't feel anything, so I try to calculate the pressure it needs and I pull it off to free my legs."

Once the sheet is off he can see his legs and then can move them,

"Now my feet, I must put them on the floor controlling the movements with my eyes. I have made up my mind. I am going to stand up. I must get my chest to tip forward, so

I have to bend my head and swing my body. The only sensation I have is a tightening in the stomach. I mustn't close my eyes. I must watch what I'm doing, all the time. The tiniest distraction—and everything crumbles."

He struggles to his feet, while from behind the Doctor watches him attentively. The Patient slowly walks forward.

"Now that I've managed to stand up, I can walk, but I can't turn round."

The Doctor turns him.

PATIENT. "If I want to keep on my feet, I have to focus on a point on the wall to know I am upright—even now when I am talking to you. And I can't do two things at once. I can stand and hold something in my hand, but if I want to walk I'm forced to look at my legs . . ."

He takes a few steps and at once he crushes the paper cup the Doctor has put in his hand.

"The doctors say, 'Neurologically, no progress.' Or else, 'You've learned to walk. Bravo!' They are right. Nothing has been achieved. I can walk today but there's no guarantee I can do so tomorrow. Every day is a mental marathon. Nothing gets recorded, there are no habits, I've only tricks and strategies. I even learned gestures to let people think I am normal."

He sits back in his chair, crossing his legs. Then he gets up again.

"Once, just once, when I was walking in the forest, I was able to look around me, listen, think, and even dream. It only lasted a few seconds, but it was marvelous to remember what it was like to be free."

Finally then, it ended with hope; the one time Ian remembers walking in the forest and being aware of what was all around him rather than of walking itself. This one short period has, alas, not recurred. "That was on the edge of New Park Farm and it's never happened again."

It was strange to hear. The poem touched me the most. I wrote it when I was depressed about my future. To see that on stage was a lot harder than if I had read it myself. Being portrayed directly was tough. I did not choke back tears, but I did reflect on my journey and how bleak things were when I wrote the poem. There seemed to be little or no opportunity ahead. Then, some years later you are in a theater as someone is reading your words back to you. It was surreal.

To be honest I was flattered by it all, who wouldn't be, and so I let some elements stand without challenging. David portrayed me sufficiently for the audience to get an idea of the condition and its consequences. But, given another chance, I would have changed bits. They used the shortest actor in the company to portray me, and so got the imagery badly wrong. My stage portrayal would have been easier and more believable with a taller actor. Come on, even Tom Cruise, with all his acting capabilities, can't do tall.

They returned to Paris for the press night. As can be imagined a new Brook play, and one in collaboration with Oliver Sacks, was big news and the theater was heaving. Ian became part of the circus. His younger brother David also came up from Marseilles on leave from the Foreign Legion.

Before the performance Marie-Hélène asked Ian to do an interview with a French radio station. Ian happily did one, then another, and a third. This made him late for supper in the theater restaurant. Eventually he sat with his brother when Marie-Hélène asked for one more interview. Ian agreed but asked if it could just be 5 minutes so he could eat before curtain up. A man came up with a microphone with the recorder being carried by his assistant. Before they started David took his watch off, placed it on the table and said in French, "Five minutes but no more." They did the interview and then David counted down the clock to zero. They asked for one more question. As David stood up, the sound man legged it, ripping the mike out the interviewer's hand. Actors are good at gesture, but a serving member of the Foreign Legion can also employ impressive body language.

Though even less of a theater man than Ian, David still loved the play, and being bilingual understood it better.

> He is a tough nut but he was touched, and quite emotional at seeing his brother portrayed on stage. Sitting together in Paris watching it, given our upbringing from the backstreets, was amazing. The vignette moved him—especially the poem.

The following day normal service resumed. Ian and David went out, round Notre Dame. They needed a pee and found an outside pissoir. It was pouring with rain, and as they stood water from the street poured over their feet. They turned to each other and laughed out loud at the nonsense of peeing into a trough while standing in a river of water. Schoolboy humor healed the intensity of the poem and the portrayal. Though Ian was grateful David had come to see it, how much better it was to share loud laughter in a flooded pissoir.

L'Homme Qui was powerful and the reactions of the audience told of its resonance with them, but Ian and Jonathan both needed to see it in English. The chance came later at The National Theatre in London, when it was performed by the same company as *The Man Who*.

Theaters and cinemas are a problem for Ian. Not only is access difficult, but once the action starts they tend to be dark. He usually gets there early and leaves late, and hopes that there will be sufficient light during the production and that his seat is secure enough for him to be able to sit without fear of falling out. He usually also wears white trainers; they are comfortable and he is used to them, but equally important they allow him to see his feet easily. But at The National he wore a dark shirt, black jacket and trousers, and matching shoes. The problem was that the auditorium was very dark too, so even with the lights on he could not really see his shoes to walk down the steps to his seat. "The theater was so dark it was difficult to get round. I managed to get down a few steps to sit next to Oliver [Sacks]. Colin Brennan, a journalist, was in the balcony with his wife and they waved. Oliver waved back and I said, 'Actually, they are waving at me.' Oliver laughed."

For Ian, seeing the whole thing in English for the first time was revelatory:

> It was mind blowing; it was a blast. It's a condition; it's something you manage on a day to day basis. Suddenly it is part of a play, doing a tour and it's at The National done by Brook. It is humbling, unbelievable. I did not expect to see myself in that situation. When I was starting to move, then stand or walk, you never expect it to see your own vignette in a play. Even watching it I found it difficult to really think it was me; it became part of a series of portrayals which were L'Homme Qui. It blows you away.

The show toured the UK and Ian saw it again in Newcastle, sitting in the front row.[3] During his vignette Ian was sitting, legs crossed, resting an elbow on his thigh as he cupped his chin in his hand, lost in thought. David Bennent was doing the same posture—exactly—on stage, art imitating nature, in real time, in front of an audience unaware of what was happening.

Its first run took 18 months as it went through France, Germany, the UK, and the USA. The reviews were almost all kind. Ian's vignette received a fair amount of attention, possibly because it was one of the longer ones and so allowed more time for people to get into his character. Paul Taylor reviewed the play for the UK newspaper *The Independent* (March 21, 1994):

The Powerlessness of Mind over Matter

A former US president used to be the butt of a cheap gag that claimed he couldn't walk and chew gum at the same time. Since this was meant to reflect on his IQ rather than on his brain condition, the Gerald Ford Syndrome is not one that is recognised by neurology. But, suppose that you were highly intelligent and yet could not walk and hold a cup at the same time, having lost all ability to move except by staring fixedly at the part of the body you wished to shift. Suppose, too, that there was no guarantee from one day to the next that you would be able to achieve even this, so that nothing remained as a habit, but had to be daily relearned as tricks and stratagems in a humiliating and exhausting mental marathon.

The irony for Ian is that the situation is still the same. It is still exhausting and still he does not know from one day to the next if he can manage.

I have a raft of movements that have been developed and that I am comfortable with. But it took an inordinate amount of time before these became trusted. My challenge now is in being able to choreograph them together into structured and managed actions such as sitting, reaching, standing, and walking. And it is the planning or sequencing that really takes the effort.

One question that crops up regularly is that having performed an action a number of times does it become automatic. Sadly, no. I have to learn every day.

Just because I did it once doesn't mean I still can. It is hard to quantify the effort required to manage the process, and as I have got older my ability to manage has diminished. It is not just the planning; it is the permanent monitoring required throughout the process to be safe. I certainly couldn't undertake some of the complex long events I used to anymore. Walking through a busy train station at rush hour would no longer be feasible, or undertaking a week's shopping at the supermarket. I have always wondered how my abilities will change as I get older. But at 60+ I am still exploring my abilities. I have recognized, more and more, that to achieve my full potential I have to be at my best. Any distraction, whether physical such as a cold or something troubling me like a family issue, diminishes my abilities.

Ian had worked so hard to stand, walk, work, and gesture to appear as others, as "normal." The play was brilliant for him in reinforcing this achievement. He was also enormously gratified that his mother lived to see such an appreciation of what he had achieved. Ian thought David Bennent portrayed him well, but he was not sure how much he had got inside him.[4] Perhaps that was just as well. Peter and his troupe were very aware of the need to portray Ian's condition and to humanize it, but avoided picking away at his privacy as well.

Most reviews were accurate but, perhaps surprisingly, one newspaper's review focused on Ian's vignette in detail suggesting it was a fable. 'If only,' as Ian says, 'If only.'

6

"THE MAN WHO LOST HIS BODY"

It had always been suspected that there were many more people like Ian and Ginette.[1] So it was not a complete surprise when Oliver Sacks sent some film from Howard Poizner's lab at Rutgers University. Howard had been studying Charles Freed, who lived in Pennsylvania and had lost proprioception at the age of 60, 7 years earlier. Jonathan got in touch with Charles and his wife Marilyn, and arranged for Ian to meet them at their home near Pittsburgh.

Charles was amazed at how long Ian had been in hospital. He explained that he had had his rehabilitation—13 weeks; that was what the insurance companies would pay for and so that now defined what rehabilitation was. Charles and Marilyn introduced Ian to their team; a big beefy physical therapist and a young occupational therapist. They explained how they had kept Charles' strength up by exercises and weights in order to prevent wasting. Now Ian had never had much wasting, maybe because his movements were more of an effort than for most people, and their emphasis on strength and muscle bulk puzzled Ian. His problem, he explained, was not power but coordination.

When they arrived, it was clear that Charles looked to Jonathan, wrongly, for a cure or for some new way of improving. Instead, Ian gave him a masterclass in how to move without touch or proprioception. Seeing Ian explain this to Charles was an eye opener to Jonathan too, since Ian covered many practical concerns in movement in a simple and accessible way. In his backyard Charles showed his "standing," with the physical therapist holding him under the arms, and with his whole body rigid. The therapist manhandled him forward one leg at a time, rocking from side to side like a stiff puppet. Each movement had uncertain shaking, ataxia, the hallmark of proprioceptive loss. After watching this Ian showed how he walked and stood. To walk he explained, to move one leg forward from a stand, you first had to contract the back muscles to lift the hip and the forward moving leg, otherwise it hit the ground. Though Charles had been upright, he had never really analysed what he needed to do himself for independent standing or walking.[2]

Ian explained he had begun by "wheelchair walking," placing one foot in front of the chair and dragging himself towards it.[3] Charles also did this, but was ataxic. Ian explained that even for this movement he controlled each foot's movement absolutely. Each and every movement had to be precise, controlled, and owned by him.

Charles showed us one of his movements on his back lawn. He transferred from wheelchair to lawn by putting his arms out on front of him and, essentially, throwing himself forward, catching most of his weight on his outstretched hands before rolling onto the ground. From low down it looked like he was parachuting out of a plane. Ian was fascinated, admiring Charles's guts, but also appalled. He would never make any movement that he could not control in its beginning, its end, and all parts in between. For him such a "ballistic" movement was not only dangerous, it was anathema; going against everything he had taught himself.[4]

Throwing a ball was another lesson, this time in how a goal can be achieved by different actions. Ian and Charles sat on the lawn, legs out in front of them, throwing a soft ball between them. Each time Charles tried to throw he moved his arm behind his shoulder, and promptly fell over backwards, since his arm weighed enough to change his center of gravity. Ian, in contrast, threw underarm by cocking the arm in front of him, allowing him to see it the whole time and avoid changing his balance. He explained that the key was to let the ball go at the right time. Charles soon learned, but was not satisfied. "That is not proper throwing." That comment underpinned an important difference between them. Ian had accepted that doing things the same way as before was no longer possible, but that with ingenuity and concentration he could find new ways.

For a few days Ian and Charles hung out, discussing movement and control and coordination rather than power. Ian taught Charles to use a metronome to entrain his movements and improve concentration, and to get into a flow. To improve his finger movements Ian had spent days and weeks making a paper clip chain. Charles tried, sitting with his arms out in front and trying to use all his fingers. Ian suggested resting his wrists on the edge of the table, to reduce the ataxia, and then to use two fingers and the thumbs as pincers, keeping the third and fourth fingers out of the way. By so reducing the degrees of freedom of the movement Charles improved in minutes.[5]

Since Ian had been working with Jonathan they had thought his experience might suit a television documentary approach. That way he could be seen and the concept of proprioception explored before a wider audience. They approached the UK's flagship science program, the BBC's *Horizon*, The editor, John Lynch, suggested a program as part of a series featuring Oliver Sacks, being filmed by Rosetta Pictures, directed by Chris Rawlence, and produced by Emma Crichton-Miller.

Chris's challenge was to reveal to an audience exactly what Ian's problem was. After all Ian had lost two of the main senses, touch and proprioception, and had recovered to an unparalleled extent. This did not impress the BBC. So, they said, he'd lost this stuff and yet no one would know to look at him; where was the program in that? You could see their point.

Through Marsha Ivins, an astronaut friend Jonathan had met through Oliver Sacks, they'd come across a NASA robot with robotic arms and fingers that moved its joints like a human. A person was put in special gloves that picked up hand movement and had infrared sensors on their elbow and shoulder joints. Then, as the person moved, so the robot did as well. The "operator" saw the robot arms in a head-mounted display. So, once rigged up, when they made a movement they saw the robot do the same, though they could not feel the robot arms. This, Chris thought, would show how Ian was in relation to his whole body the whole time; he intended movement, saw it happen, but could not feel it. The film crew arranged a trip to Houston.

Thanks to Marsha, once at NASA the group was able to see not just the robot but the whole facility. WET-F, the Weightless Environment Training Facility, was a giant sunken pool in which there was a submerged mock-up of the Space Shuttle's payload bay. Astronauts in their suits were swimming around practicing fixing things under the gaze of their trainers. Ian was fascinated. He asked how they taught the astronauts. The trainer replied that they explained what the task was and then gave each astronaut some time to work out how they would like to do it; then they helped each astronaut to do it in his or her own way. Ian nodded appreciatively; that was how rehabilitation should be too. He was fascinated, "Their mantra was practice, practice, practice, which I could associate with."

Marsha conducted a tour of Building 9A, a huge space where they had mock-ups of the Space Shuttle, the Space Station, and all sorts of other big toys for procedural training in ingress and egress and for orbit "choreography"—learning to move most efficiently while doing complex tasks in a small space. She led everyone up to the tiny door of the Shuttle mock-up. Ian managed to get in, but alas could not climb up to the flight deck.[6]

> Thanks to Marsha, we were able to explore much more than most guests. Here was I climbing around the Shuttle; absolutely astounding; I loved every moment of it. Never in a million years would I have dreamed this was possible. I remember having a long chat with Dan Barry, and the next time I saw him was on the BBC News as he circled the earth in the Shuttle. Quite an experience for a butcher's boy with an unusual neuropathy.

The robot was in another building, but before this, in one room there was a mysterious large metal block suspended on wires at body height, with each side measuring around a meter. On one side was a steering wheel. The block could be made to behave as though it had a variety of masses or gravitational forces upon it. It could, for instance, be made to move as though it had a large mass in zero gravity to simulate docking equipment in space.

Perhaps we were all a bit blasé, but we did not brief Ian about how special this block was. He stood up, held the wheel, and gave it a shove. It moved, and then just carried on moving slowly, like a boat across a lake. Whether Ian expected it to resist, once started, or to spring back was unclear, but suddenly he had a problem. Standing up and holding on, he was now being pulled by a force with a completely unexpected behavior. When he stands, to make sure he is upright, he looks at fixed spots in the surrounding world, a door frame, window, tree stump, or whatever, which are stationary and allow him to calibrate his position in relation to the world. It is the lack of these cardinal points on a ship or plane, where everything he can see is moving in relation to gravity, that prevents him moving during a flight. Here, his visual fix on the block had failed and it was behaving in a way he could not decode. Unable to decide whether to hold on or let go, his eyes were flicking from block, to floor, to side wall, as he tried to work out what was happening. Immediately the engineers stopped the block and Ian recovered:

> The machine and I just didn't get on. The problem was that I was standing directly in front of the block, and apart from extreme peripheral vision there was very limited feedback. It was a nightmare and I just couldn't master it. Totally frustrating, but great fun.

Next was the robot. Oliver was first to have a go, and had a great time playing. Chris filmed as Oliver explained how he could see the robot arm and move it, but had no sense of touch, and how curious that was. Thus far the analogy with Ian held. Then it was Ian's turn. He was rigged up and, once anchored and strapped into the chair, put on the head-mounted display (HMD), so that he saw the robot arms but not his own, nor his body. This was when the analogy broke down. When Oliver was in the device he could move and see the robot while also feeling his own arms and hands. It did not matter that he could not see them since he knew where they were through proprioception. Ian was able to move his hands and arms, and to close and open his fingers by seeing the robot movements, but in the HMD he had no idea where his arms were. The only way he could establish this was to move them quickly, which gave a hunting, shuddery movement to the robot arms as they caught up. Though the analogy between us and Ian was not exact in the robot,

Ian was able to move the robot fingers and hands well, even though he was a little unsure where they were. But even this became easier, and when someone suggested Ian should pick up an egg, to demonstrate just how sensitive the robot fingers were, Ian was happy to try.

A table was placed in front of the robot, eggs found, and after the engineers had protected their robot hand in a Marigold glove, filming started. Sure enough Ian managed to move the robot arms to the egg, put the fingers round it, and then, gripping slightly, lift the unbroken egg. One problem for Ian was what to do next, so he put the egg down again.[7]

> Working with the robot was a massively challenging task, and I was working at my limit for sure. What researchers tend to forget is that subjects feel they have to "perform", and that's not good for research or the subject. I like to think I can generally cope with this well, but this event was different. There had been so much hype, and as I understood it the filming was to be a key element in the program. Yeah, so no pressure then.
>
> With the visor on I essentially lost all reference to me, and found it hard to concentrate on anything other than not falling out of the chair. The so-called simple tasks were not simple for me, although I did eventually become more competent.
>
> Picking up the egg with the robotic hand was a blast, and I even got a round of applause. One of the technicians told me I was the first to do this so I was feeling pleased with myself. The moment of glory was short lived, I learned later they had small servos to control finger grip. A vivid image remains of the lab technician who sat the whole time we were there with his hand over a 'cut off' button if we were about to damage their very expensive toy.

Jonathan too, soon learned to move slowly when it was his turn; there was a delay between his movement and the robot's which, when seen, was nauseating if he moved too fast. Passing a wrench from hand to hand was curiously and unexpectedly fun. Jonathan became completely absorbed and then realized, a minute or so later, that if he dropped the mole wrench, which was quite heavy, it would land on his leg. He had become completely embodied in the robot.

Everyone had the same strong illusion. Ian remembers:

> In a very short space of time I was embodied; the robot and I were one. When, some 20 feet away, a trolley was pushed towards the robot, and as I was wearing the visor, I responded immediately and took evasive action to protect myself, or my "new self" as seen through the visor. A surreal and spooky moment. I thought it could be explained because I rely upon my sight so heavily and I was "seeing" the world through the robot. But apparently this phenomenon happens to everyone. How strange that after all the years of happily inhabiting our bodies we can so quickly let it go and become entwined with another object.

Oliver experienced the same, as had the engineers. We are embodied in what we move and see moving. Our body ownership can—perhaps surprisingly—shift rapidly into a robot.[8]

It was soon after this filming trip that Chris decided that the program might be better as a stand-alone one with Ian and Jonathan. Oliver was filming a short series on different neurological conditions, and his great strength was to convey the experience of those, whether with Tourette's, autism, color blindness, or Williams' syndrome, who find it difficult to convey their experience themselves. Ian was more than able to portray his condition and Jonathan could say something about the neuroscience. As Chris said, "We just felt that it was Ian and Jonathan's quest rather than Oliver's."

All the filming with Oliver, including the NASA tapes, had to be cut. Instead Chris and Emma skillfully combined an unveiling narrative with the necessary scientific explanation, in what was called "The Man Who Lost His Body."[9]

The film opened with Charles, in slow motion, "parachuting" from his wheelchair onto his lawn. The voice-over explained that his problem was not paralysis but loss of proprioception, the hidden sixth sense of movement and position sense (though of course cutaneous touch was also lost). Proprioception was "so basic that most are unaware that we have it." Ian walked and Charles crawled across his lawn. Ian was concerned about this stark emphasis of their difference but, given the BBC executive's concern about making Ian's recovery visible, it was necessary.

Watching the film again, 15 years later, Ian's comments were all particular, about the movements made. For example, he was amazed at how much Charles wobbled as he fell out the chair, with his weight on his right hip:

> That fall is not controlled. I would never do that. I would have practiced it and broken it down into elements and made each more stable. He is trusting to luck and good fortune.

The film then cut to Herb Schaumberg, a professor of neurology in New York who first described the sensory neuronopathy syndrome, expressing astonishment that Ian was walking. "I assumed he would be in a chair. It's the sort of thing you expect to happen at Lourdes." Ian then recited his poem, *Living Death*, which Brook had also used, as we saw him lying on his old hospital bed. This part, revisiting his worst times, could not have been easy. Ian continued:

> It's not until now, filming, that—it's like a lid on a box one does never even open. It was very bleak and I was very frightened.

Seeing the film again triggered memories of filming and of the early days:

I normally don't look back. I forgot the days lying on a bed able to do nothing, thinking how on earth to move. It made me realize how much my illness had affected others. A big motivation to me then, and now, is not wanting to feel guilty about asking others to help me. All disabilities have an impact on those around them.[10]

In Jersey they had tried to get me to walk. I had a pajama top but no bottom, so they found a nappy-like thing and put it on me, with three pins. Then three physios assisted, one each side and one on the floor positioning my feet as I was marched along. I will never forget the indignity of being walked in the middle of the ward in front of everyone else. I was completely humiliated and totally embarrassed. There appeared to be no thought about what they were doing personally, emotionally, or morally. In those days I was not vocal and so said nothing. But it made me realize what I had become, with my mobility stolen.

The film followed him to the Wessex Neurological Centre in Southampton and then to Odstock Hospital for rehabilitation. He was walking along a gloomy, empty corridor and then into a room full of broken wheelchairs; this was his old ward: "I fought long and hard not to go into a wheelchair and I was arrogant, bloody minded, and difficult, they remember me so well I must have been very difficult." The film cut to Ian on a bed again, puzzling how to move. The voice-over explained that eventually Ian began to realize that the solution might be that if he could visualize a movement he could make it happen. Still on the bed he related:

I remember tensing the tummy muscles, and folding up in the middle and never getting anywhere. After a lot of practice and effort I learned a technique to lift the head forward, move the shoulders, and then sit up, I remember vividly the first time, I was so euphoric I lost all control and almost fell out of bed. That simple act of sitting up was the key to movement if it was to be controlled for the rest of my life. That I would have to plan it before I did it, structure it in my mind, work my way through it, and that's how it is today. It hasn't changed.

Looking again recently, Ian remembered;

I learned by a hunch, or more likely by accident; I fell into a strategy that worked. I placed everything visually, legs apart and arms by the side, and then curling up from the head and with a flick of the shoulders I could roll up. It was only afterwards that I analyzed what I did.

The film then cut to Ian and Charles on a lawn, chatting and throwing a ball. Rewatching the film, Ian was fascinated to see how he sat:

My right arm is locked round my right leg with the knee bent, so I looked cool. But it was a con trick; then I could only gesture with the left arm. When I sat on the beach later it was the same, and when leaning against a shack at the hospital. This assuming a pose, or creating an image, is essentially a façade to look normal, acting. But over the years they have become more accomplished, more natural, they are now me.

As he caught the ball his arms went back and, as they did, his spine arched back as well. Some movements were apparently automatic, or at least not attended to:

> I was thinking about catching the ball; the spine moved itself in compensation.[11]

The next sequence followed Ian walking through a shopping center into a greengrocer's shop, to relate how he had left hospital and returned to the world. As he walked, Ian explained, "I would have to scan the ground ahead, not immediately but about 6 or 8 feet ahead, so I am planning all the time. I am aware of where I am going to put my feet so I am not compromising myself." He does not let someone walk the other way between him and wall. Later there was a girl outside the greengrocer—Ian could remember the sequence:

> I was tired and only reacted to the guy walking towards me near the end of my ability to correct and move. In contrast I saw the girl way before and was avoiding her and plotting where she might go.

As he walked, Ian explained in a prerecorded piece, that, "An athlete will train and train for a competition, and that is their peak, what they strive for. I work at my peak every day. It sounds dramatic, and almost over the top, but it is not. I live at the edge every day, all day, there is no leeway."

The voice-over related how the simplest of actions can tip him over. Shopping becomes an exercise in mechanics. In the film Ian picked up a vegetable:

> Swedes are an odd thing; sometimes they can be really heavy and sometimes light. Picking one up can do a lot for my balance. I will get into a safe position for my feet, freeze my legs rigidly, then I know they will not move around a lot, freeze the upper torso so it is rigid and then I can start handing off my bodily frame other arm movements. But I have to be aware that it is a heavy object and the laws of physics say that a heavy object lifted out-stretched from a narrow base and you're going to topple over. I have to think what picking up that object is going to do to my narrow framework.

The voice-over continued "for the next 10 years Ian went his own way. College, Civil Service, marriage." Felice explained about Mavis. Next, Ian is walking along in front of a laid out Saturn V rocket at NASA, just after a thunderstorm, in strong sunlight against the stormy sky. Given his condition his rhythm and grace are beautiful. Watching again he said:

> I have done millions of steps, but I know what goes into them. I cannot do them unthinkingly, automatically. Knowing precisely where I am at all times is essential in

everything I do. I tend to lumber along at a certain rhythm. I could never run, nor could I suddenly freeze, since it would be unstable in a vulnerable posture.[12]

Next the film moved to science: "Ian kept away from specialists, but then he was introduced to Jonathan Cole." They were shown sitting in a seaside café drinking tea. Then there was a sequence comparing similarities between Ian's condition and those of Marsha Ivins in space. She explained that she has reduced proprioception in space and so how she has to think about movement when she goes up and, once adapted to zero gravity, when she returns to Earth. "We take gravity for granted. We take for granted how far to pick up [our] feet when walking for example. For a while when returning from space to 1g we forget that."[13] The film showed some shots of astronauts just after they had returned from a mission. They were walking awkwardly and concentrating on what they did. Marsha continued:

> Whatever that sequence is between hip, knee, and ankle, they all go in a certain order, I find for an hour or two after coming back that there is a joint that forgets that order, so I had to be careful and think about each limb. When I come back if someone's going to hug me, like Ian, I have to get braced for it, or I am not sure where I am going. You have to learn to move in zero g and that takes a long time.

The film then moved to a very different area, gesture, and to Chicago where Professor David McNeill studied Ian's use of gesture. Ian watched a cartoon (of Sylvester the Cat and Tweety) and then subsequently had to relay what happened in the story, allowing David to analyze his gesture in minute detail, millisecond by millisecond. David also isolated Ian from his gesture by using a screen below his neck so he could not see his arms and hands.[14]

Watching all this again, Ian said:

> I was not happy, just trying to look happy. Look where my eyes go. When describing gestures, I was again hinged at the elbow [arms by his body, resting on the chair arm]. Then I could do throwaways [gestures with little attention]. But see, I did not use both arms together, it was one or the other. I would put one down and pick the other up. I left one on my lap in between, and the other on the chair arm, to avoid a mid-air collision.
>
> It is irrefutable to me. I am thinking about it and presenting myself and performing. I am intimidated so trying to look cool, so I crossed my legs in this shot, to appear casual. Earlier both feet were on the ground. But with legs crossed I would only use one arm to gesture; otherwise it is not safe; two arms need two legs. I had spent years building up movements which did not look contrived and yet which were, and I was concerned he would see through them. I knew I was performing and could see it on film.

The film concluded with a functional imaging experiment at The National Hospital for Nervous Diseases and Neurosurgery in London. With Richard

Frakowiak, Chris Frith, Daniel Wolpert, and research fellow Bal Athwal they devised a simple experiment; touching each finger to the thumb with feedback from a video screen. Then they were able compare brain activations in four conditions; when Ian moved and saw his finger move, when he moved but saw a still hand, when he had a still hand and saw that hand still, and lastly when his hand was still but he saw his recorded hand moving. They then compared Ian's brain activations with those of six controls (Jonathan was one).[15]

In the most interesting condition, Ian moving without being able to see his hand move, he activated an area of right orbito-frontal cortex more than controls, reflecting his need for top-down control or mental concentration, even for a simple movement. He alone also activated an area of the occipito-parietal cortex. To move without feedback he has to concentrate on moving, and what he thinks about is visualizing what he is doing. He has always said that he uses visualization to move; now there were brain imaging data in support of this. He was closing the open control loop for

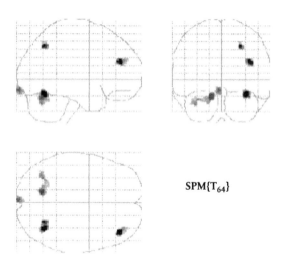

SPM{T_{64}}

Fig. 6.1. Composite PET scans during finger movement without informative vision. The figure shows the brain from the right (top left), behind (top right), and from above. The dark areas represent areas of increased blood flow, and hence higher brain activity, in Ian compared with six control subjects while they moved their thumb to their fingers (left hand) repetitively at 1 Hz (in time to a metronome) while watching a video of their own hands being still, i.e. moving without being able to see their hands moving. Ian activated an area of pre-frontal cortex more than control subjects, possibly reflecting his greater conscious control of this movement, and of occipito-parietal cortex, possibly reflecting his method of moving without vision, using conscious visual imagery of his moving hand in the absence of direct vision. He also activated areas of cerebellum, lower down in the composite scan.

movement by entraining his intention by visualization (Fig. 6.1). Several areas of the cerebellum were also activated on both sides, which is more difficult to explain.

The whole film concluded with Ian walking through his beloved New Forest, camera and tripod in hand, to photograph deer. Ian had the last word:

> I have occasionally thought to myself why go through all this? Why make it difficult for myself? There is an awful lot of effort just to be mobile. I do not know how long I will keep that up. Had it affected me more recently, I might have been more mature and accepting of disability perhaps. Society is more accepting too. I might not have felt the need to work so hard.

Ian's first thoughts on looking back 15 years later were of how tired he must have been during the walking sequences and of his posture and gestures at the time. His best memories were of filming and the fun he and Jonathan had off camera with Chris Rawlence and cameraman Chris Morphet.

"The Man Who Lost His Body" was seen by around 1.6 million viewers at the time in the UK, and has been televised round the world and is now available on the internet. One result was a minor deluge of people who got in contact to say they had a similar condition.[16] Ian and Jonathan met a few of these "Ian-a-likes"; some had sensory loss which was less severe but still devastating for them. Ian helped them as best he could with tips about how to move and advice about what level of functioning they could maintain.

Chris and the team had thought long and hard about the title for the documentary and the one they decided on had appeared rather sensational. Ian was not keen on it, but towards the end of the filming sequences, during the PET experiment, it suddenly became appropriate. He had to spend 2 hours on his back, in a scanner, without vision of his body. Jonathan was with him the whole time reassuring him that his body and legs were OK. But for Ian, not seeing his body for that length of time was profoundly disquieting:

> It's very difficult to explain. I got in panic mode, not knowing where I was, or if I was safe; I asked Jonathan a number of times, "Are my legs OK? Is my arm OK?"

Ian is usually very adept at deflecting attention from the precariousness of his condition. The experiment had not been designed to reveal how necessary vision was for his embodiment and his sense of self, but at the end of the experiment, and for that brief period, without feeling from his body and without visual reassurance, he had no disguise and he really was a man who had lost his body.

GOING PARABOLIC

The Pull of Zero Gravity

On Thursday, April 26, 2007, Stephen Hawking, the Lucasian Professor of Mathematics at Cambridge University, experienced microgravity weightlessness on a parabolic flight. He was, it was reported, the first person with a disability to experience weightlessness.[1] Ian was amused; he had flown on the Vomit Comet a decade before. For the final sequence of the BBC *Horizon* film Chris Rawlence had planned to film Ian weightless. Having filmed Marsha Ivins describing her experience aboard the Space Shuttle and how, without gravity, she had shared some of Ian's experiences on the ground, cutting her footage with Ian's when weightless would have wrapped the film on a high. But seeing a chance for some science as well, the team approached Jim Lackner and his assistant Paul DiZio at Brandeis University, Boston. A world expert in the neuroscience of microgravity, Jim suggested that they should go to his lab for preliminary experiments before moving to NASA's operation at their airfield, Ellington Field Joint Reserve Base, in Houston.

Ian was up for this:

> I trust Jonathan with research projects, to keep me safe and that it is good science. But my first thought was that this would be fun. You are very rarely, as someone disabled, put in such a radical position, experiencing new things and pushing yourself. It was also so bloody exciting. I used to say to friends, "I am going parabolic," and they would say, "What's that?" and I would say, "Remember *Apollo 13*? That is how they filmed it." The friends could go along with that. I had kudos; I was cool.
>
> It is boring being disabled, with so few opportunities to do something so bizarre. I also thought that, since I was valuable as a guinea pig, they would not let me die. I have always said my journey was so long, and my hold on normal function so tenuous, that I would not put it at risk. This was one of the few times when I just went for it. I could not predict what it would be like and so would have to adapt at the time. This was fun—bloody amazing fun—and you don't get many chances like that.

Before they went, however, they had to persuade NASA to allow Ian to fly. Jim suggested saying as little as possible to avoid fuss. Slowly, however, the NASA medics started taking more and more interest. Could we explain exactly what Ian's disability was? (Not easy.) How would he evacuate the plane in a hurry? (Badly, Ian said, but he was ready to take the risk.) We persisted. NASA then said they needed a full pilot's medical, with a medical, eye, and ear testing and decompression training. If he passed all those then they might allow him to fly.

At the medical Ian was found to have high blood pressure and was put on treatment. NASA were not impressed and said the blood pressure had to be down before he could fly. Next were eye and ear tests, which required a trudge up to London. These tests passed, next was decompression training.

The weightless flight plane, or KC135, flies in parabolas, between 34,000 and 23,000 feet, with 25 seconds of weightlessness at the top of its arc and then 50 seconds of 1.8g as it climbs back up again. The NASA flights have four sets of ten parabolas. For most of the time people are doing various experiments moving around in the plane's fuselage and so are away from the emergency oxygen. In case of decompression they have a few seconds to get to their seats and their oxygen mask, before passing out and then dying (unless someone else puts their mask on). They needed a certificate covering the decompression training required to alert them to their first symptoms of cerebral hypoxia. Some people feel lightheaded, others lose color vision. One astronaut was slightly skeptical; her first symptom was unconsciousness, and she relied completely on her colleagues to put her mask on.

Ian, Chris Morphet, the cameraman, and Jonathan turned up at RAF Luffenham, near Stamford in Lincolnshire. It was opened in 1940 and then, after the war, was home to fighters and then ballistic missiles. In 1960 part of the RAF School of Aviation Medicine was moved there with a "state-of-the-art" decompression chamber. Despite all this it seemed that little had changed since the 1940s. Miles from anywhere, it was an anonymous collection of low, drab buildings.

They were led to a big room with, in the center, a large metal tube with portholes; the decompression chamber. It had seats either side with room for a dozen or so inside. Ian found it all excellent:

> We had Biggles hats, goggles, and oxygen masks; it was a big adventure. I was amused that Chris, a wonderful cameraman, was a bit nervous. The trainer started talking about the number of brain cells which die at high altitude and Chris went a pale.

Word of Ian's condition had got around, and that if he was hypoxic he would fall off the bench because he wouldn't be able to think straight. There was quite a crowd of scientists looking in through the portholes. Suddenly there was a noise like a bath emptying; the air was changed from the composition at sea level to that found at

34,000 feet, reducing the amount of oxygen in the air by 83%. We had been warned this might trigger mass belching and farting; mercifully sphincters held tight. Then they worked their way round the group, taking off the masks, two by two, until each person had early symptoms of hypoxia. This was not an ideal way to simulate unexpected decompression.

Ian's mask was removed, with several instructors close by. He was not happy doing mental arithmetic. By the time he'd finished arguing, they put the mask back on:

> The hypoxic test was amusing. You realize how vulnerable you appear to others when you see a large number of white-coated people looking into the chamber waiting for you to fall out the chair. I have always had an aversion to maths but love arguing. My dying breath will probably involve an argument with someone over something trivial.

Ian had no symptoms either. Fun, yes, and necessary, but completely useless otherwise.

All the time Jim and Jonathan were working on NASA, convincing them that Ian was not really disabled and that he could walk on and off the plane OK. We did not tell them he would not be able to walk at all once it was in flight, but they never asked. He was on the flight.[2]

The Ashton Graybiel Spatial Orientation Laboratory at Brandeis University, outside Boston, researches aspects of motion sickness, the perception of human body orientation, and the effects of varying force environments on movement, posture, and balance. Many of these interests coalesce around the vestibular system of the inner ear. Their research has relevance to problems in aeronautics and astronautics as well as some clinical ones.

Be that as it may, what Ian remembers are the steps and steep ramp at the front of the building, so they went in via the basement, down a longer, shallower ramp. The lab was also in the basement, without windows, with ten or so rooms full of equipment. For a neurophysiologist it was a cave of delights, with so many different ways to make someone sick. There were chairs in which people could be spun in several planes thus inducing vertigo, nausea, and often sickness. Another experiment, the optokinetic drum, involved a large turntable on which someone walked (with a horizontal bar at waist height to hold), surrounded by vertical stripes from top to bottom. The drum, turntable, and stripes could all be rotated independently, and if the stripes were rotated backwards they induced the illusion that even though the subject was walking forwards on the turntable they thought they were reversing.

However, one of the main areas was the large rotating room. Twenty-two feet across and mounted on a World War II German gun turret motor, the room could spin fast enough to give a force at the peripheral wall of around 4g. Ian remembers:

> The spinning room was surreal. I sat in a chair right in the middle and made movements of the hand while we were being spun at various speeds.

Ian was asked to move his finger from one place close to him on a table out to another spot, both illuminated, in the dark. He sat in the center of the rotation so that as he moved outwards his arm was subject to sheering Coriolis forces, forcing it off line to the side. This force only becomes apparent during movement and is proportional to the velocity of movement. After making a movement to the required spot, and missing it to the left, one assumes (because the arm does not go where one asks it to) that some external agent must be acting. One soon learns to compensate for this and hit the target, and when the rotation stops one overshoots the other way, showing motor learning. Jonathan and the Brandeis team were interested in how Ian might approach this without proprioception. With his eyes shut Ian did not learn to compensate, as expected, but with his eyes open he learned pretty quickly. In fact his way of reducing the Coriolis force effect was to stiffen his arm during its reach, so overcoming the sideways sheer. One problem was that while it could be measured that Ian improved with visual feedback it was not possible to demonstrate how he did it since his stiffness could not easily be measured.

> In the Coriolis force chamber I chose to stiffen my arm to hit the target. It was the first strategy I tried and it worked. I doubt, having been set a target, that I would not develop a strategy, the desire and need are now automatic; not to apply one would make me less accurate, and I am extremely competitive. If you show me a target I will try to hit it my way. Even if you said relax the arm, if I was inaccurate doing this, then I would stiffen. That is what I do.

In experiments the idea is to devise a task beyond such adaptation, or to measure the stiffness of the arm in various conditions, which here the team failed to do. During some of these attempts Jonathan sat at the outside of the room, enjoying the greatest g force, throwing a tennis ball up and trying to catch it as it sped away. What surprised him was just how hard it is to raise one's head or arm against a force of 4g. Far harder, in fact, than lifting a weight in the gym, which makes the arm similarly heavy. It was as though, automatically, the nervous system had made the arm stiffer with the increased g force, just as Ian had done cognitively. It was clear that altered gravitational fields do odd things to movement and the perception of action.

Whilst at Brandeis Ian also remembers an incident with a can of Coke:

I made an arrogant statement sitting with Jim. I had asked for a drink and he came back with a can of Coke and handed it to me. I opened it and he said he was worried since he wasn't sure if he might have been expected to open it for me. My response was dismissive, along the lines that I was not completely incapable, and as long as I think the action through and plan I can manage most things. I remember thinking afterwards that I must have seemed rude and arrogant. Jim is one of the very few researchers I would return to without question; an absolute gentleman and consummate researcher.

We were all in a burger place and I asked Jim what we were doing the next day. Before he had a chance to explain, Jonathan stopped him. I must admit I get a bit of a buzz winding Jonathan up by asking seemingly "innocent" questions to researchers knowing that they shouldn't really answer me.

The more experiments Ian has done, the more it has become evident just how analytical he is. Given information about an experiment Ian will find a way of planning it. The better approach is to give him very little information and then, if necessary, give him more feedback and ideas later on. The trick is to work with him to get the right level of each. The opposite problem, that he cannot work out how to do a task at all and therefore will not attempt it, has only ever occurred once, and not during an experiment for which Jonathan was responsible.

A PhD student, Eli, was doing an experiment on the stability of standing. He had shown that when someone stands on a board which measures their natural wobble, if they just touch a stable external object with an outstretched finger, and even though they gain no support from it, their stability increases since it gives an additional point of reference in relation to the world. Eli was uncertain whether this would reduce Ian's sway, or if the mental effort of moving his hand to the point while standing would be an additional task and so lead to more wobble. The results suggested the latter; Ian was less stable using the extra point, unlike control subjects.

Ian also did one more experiment in Boston. The "turn and reach," as the name implies, was designed to study sensorimotor control and adaptation of active torso rotation, arm movement, and combinations thereof. Ian stood at a table cut out at waist level so that he was almost surrounded by it. He was asked to reach to the left or right, to touch a spot on the table with his finger, as fast as possible. The targets were positioned cunningly so he could not reach them by moving his arm alone but had to rotate his shoulders and hips as well. The researchers plotted the movement of his hands, shoulders, and hips using infrared markers and so tracked his rotation and coordination. Ian seemed to do this task in a near normal fashion by simultaneously moving his arm, shoulders, and hips; either he had learned this, or the reach and turn movement was still present as a motor program:

> I know how far I can reach with my arm and saw how far I needed to turn. I froze my legs and hips and had assessed how much latitude I had as I was getting into position. The board came up to my waist, so I could not see my feet; not a good position to be in for sure. To coordinate movement of my arm and shoulders and hips I planned ahead. My feedback of where I was in the world was visual, from the wall and the table. To twist my upper body without a visual link to below the waist was very hard, and I had to have a plan of campaign. Was I safe, how far could I move, could I use the structure for support, listen for any unusual sensations or pain, was there a chair to fall back into, what was my "get out safe" strategy, was everything OK? I could see and assess a lot with my peripheral vision as well. I put a picture in my head to make it happen. I was already planning the stop before I got there. I built up an expectation and looked for clues to keep me safe and manage the task. This was not a simple one.

Though in most experiments Ian has performed scientists have avoided giving Ian feedback or practice, the main purpose of going to Boston was for Ian to do another task he was actually trained to do by repetition and without vision; to make a simple flexion/extension movement of the elbow when sitting down. Then this same experiment could be done in zero gravity to plot how gravity influenced the unfolding of this simple learned program. To make sure he was accurate in making these reaches Ian practiced with and without vision for hours, the opposite of the usual procedure. This time the idea was to over-train Ian to see the effect of changes in gravity on his performance.

In addition to running this experiment on the KC135, Jim and Paul also had three others Ian was not to do. In one, subjects were asked to do deep and shallow knee bends and judge how deep they felt; in the second, subjects had to reach with their finger to touch between two places on a table. Performances were tracked by motion-sensitive cameras that picked up signals from sensors on the subjects' hands and bodies. In the final experiment, "sticks," subjects were handed one end of a stick and, without seeing it, had to move it up and down to judge how long it was from its weight and inertia. The sticks were balanced oddly in terms of their weight distribution. Jim was interested in how people would make this judgment in different gravitational fields, beginning in Boston at 1g and then moving to Houston for zero and 1.8g.

Ian's chair and the equipment for the knee bend and table reach experiments were all positioned next to each other in a line. Once we had done the preliminaries at Brandeis, two of Jim's lab crew put the kit and the motion-capture device on a truck and drove it, over 2 days and nights, down to Houston, reassembling it across the fuselage of the KC135 plane in exactly the same layout as in the lab. The precision and efficiency with which they did all this was brilliant. Ian and the others flew

ILLUSTRATIONS

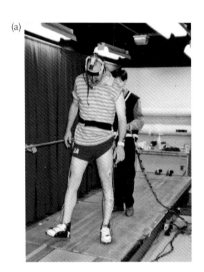

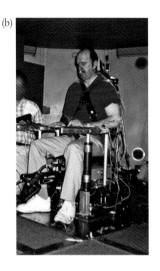

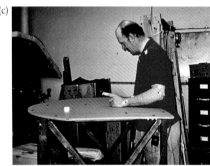

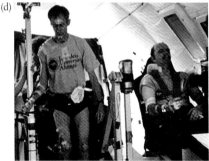

Illustration 1. Ian during experiments.

(a) On the catwalk in Laval University, Quebec, to investigate his attention towards walking. (b) In the circulating chamber at Brandeis University, Boston, for experiments on reaching during Coriolis forces, 1998. (c) Ian at the table for the turn and point experiment, Brandeis University, Boston, 1998. (d) Ian and Jonathan in KC135, the "Vomit Comet, Houston, 1998 (NASA). (e) Gait study, Aalborg, Denmark, 2007. (f) Magnetoencephalography, Helsinki, Finland, 2009. (g) Study of grasping, Birmingham, UK, 2012. (h) Study on reaching, University College London, 2013.

(e)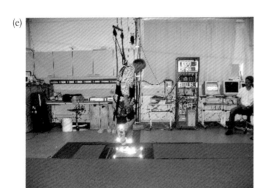

(f)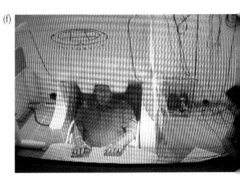

(g)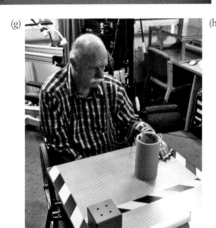

(h)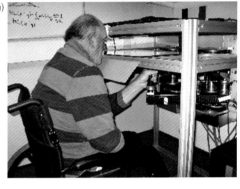

Illustration 1. Continued.

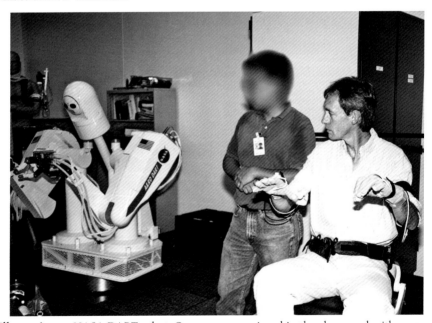

Illustration 2. NASA DART robot. Once you were rigged in the gloves and with sensors on your arms, the robot moved as you moved and you saw the robot's arms in the head-mounted display via cameras in the robot's eyes, 1997 (NASA photo).

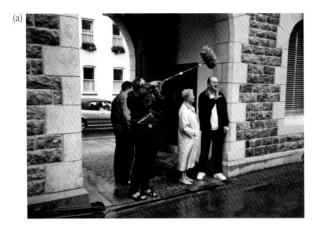

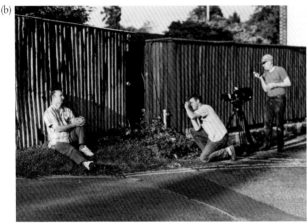

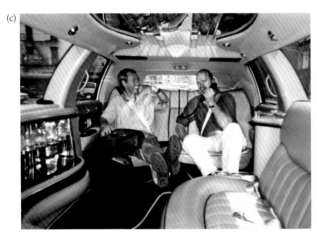

Illustration 3. The romance of filming.

(a) Ian and Felice standing on a busy road in Jersey, in the rain, looking across at his old hospital ward, 1997. (b) Ian resting in between filming in the grounds of Salisbury Hospital. Chris Rawlence, the director, is taking the still photo and Chris Morphet, the cameraman, is measuring the light before starting filming. Ian was tired, but still playing to the camera, 1997. (c) Ian and Jonathan while filming in New York, 1997.

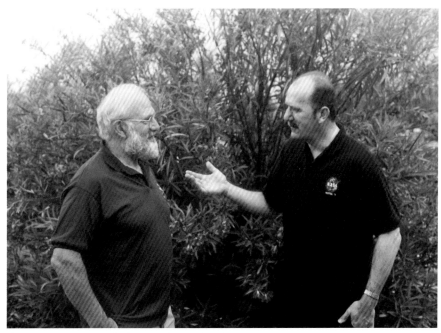

Illustration 4. Ian and Oliver Sacks, in Florida, 1997.

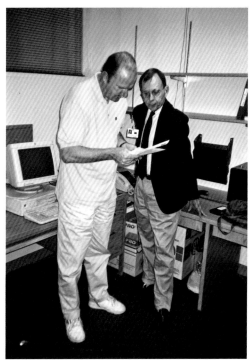

Illustration 5. Ian and Herb Schaumburg, New York City, 1997.

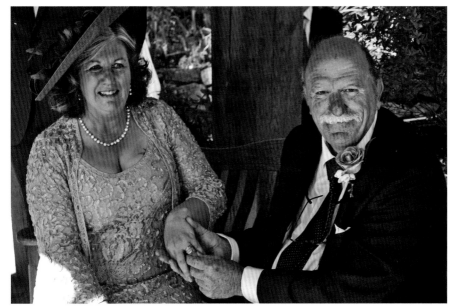

Illustration 6. Ian and Brenda at their wedding, 2013.

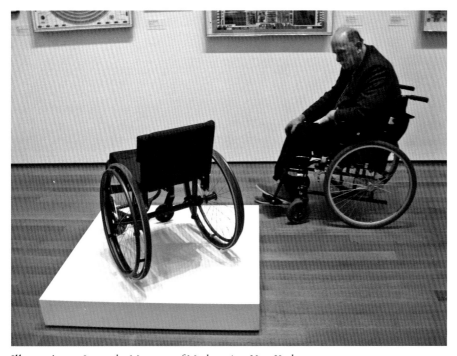

Illustration 7. Ian at the Museum of Modern Art, New York, 2013.

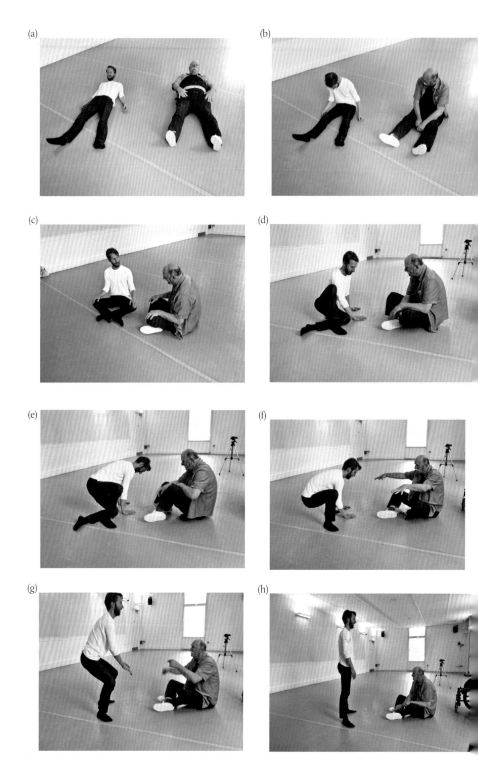

Illustration 8. Ian instructing Matthias Sperling how to stand up for Siobhan Davies' and Matthias' *Manual*, 2014 (composite).

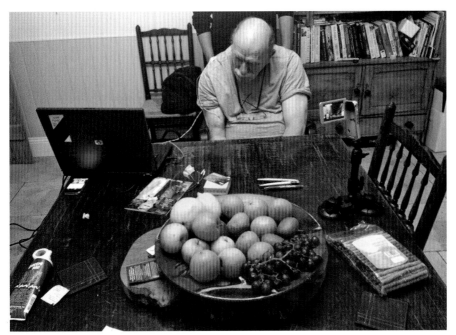

Illustration 9. Ian during a Kohnstamm experiment in his kitchen, 2013.

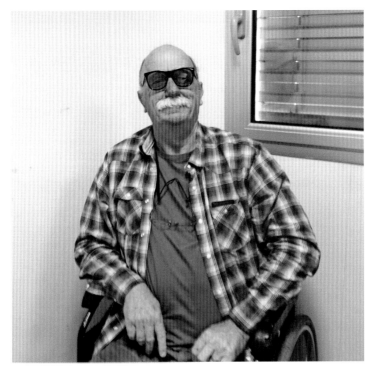

Illustration 10. Ian at CNRS, Marseilles, during an experiment on perception while using prism glasses, 2013.

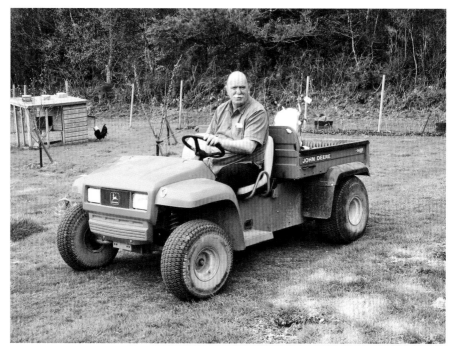

Illustration 11. Ian at home on his Gator buggy.

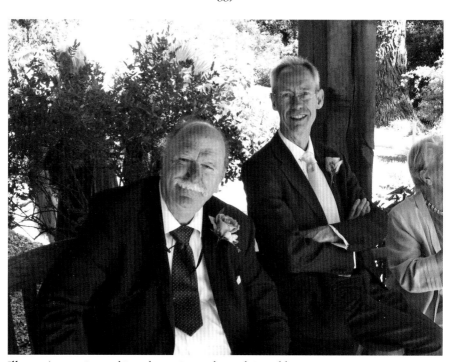

Illustration 12. Ian and Jonathan at Ian and Brenda's wedding.

down to Houston to be put up in luxurious apartments.[3] There was one last hurdle. Ian went off to have his blood pressure taken again; NASA had always said that if it was not down the day before the flight he could not go. Thankfully all was well.

Ellington Field Joint Reserve Base is on the southeast side of Houston. Ian and the others stepped out of the car onto the tarmac at the side of the runway. On one side was a huge, fat transport plane, "The Guppy," while every so often a NASA pilot would take off in a small, piercingly loud plane. The air smelt of fuel, rubber, and testosterone:

> It was fabulous schoolboy stuff. We parked on the apron and got out. It was baking hot and in front of us were these amazing planes for transporting aircraft wings. One suddenly got a sense of what would happen. It was so exciting. I remember being told to sit down, shut up, look casual, and avoid NASA's gaze.

The pre-flight instructions were in a small building next to the runway; until then Ian had not been nervous. There were two massive photos of the KC135, a modified Boeing 727, on the wall; in one it was pointing 45 degrees up and in the other 45 degrees down. These images were strangely disturbing; until then Ian had not really thought what the plane actually did during the flight, and finding out was not reassuring. One pony-tailed man in another party wore a T-shirt that read, "Actually, I *am* a rocket scientist."

> The purpose of the pre-brief was to familiarize us with the plane's emergency procedures. The oxygen masks and life jackets were under the seats. In the NASA video a man tried valiantly to take them from beneath his seat, remove the packaging, and put them on. It took so long pony-tail muttered. "They should call the video 'Kiss your ass goodbye.'"

At the end of the instruction it was announced cheerfully that the KC135 was not an IATA recognized flight and so any travel insurance would not be valid. Jonathan had anticipated this and arranged insurance through a friend who was an underwriter at Lloyds. Ian was worried that he would be sick and disgrace himself:

> It was hot and we were wearing the green zoot suits. I could not walk with the big black boots they wanted us to wear, so wore my usual shoes. Janna, one of the researchers, was taping electrodes to my finger when she carped on the cost of the tape. I said she needed to use more since I would sweat and it would come off. 'Do you know how much it costs?' she said. I said compared with how much it cost to get to Houston it was not much.

Out they trooped, zoot suited and with electrodes here, there, and everywhere, to the plane waiting outside. Black thunder clouds rolled in. Ian asked if that would delay us. No, they said, we'd fly through that. And they did; they were not normal pilots.

Entry to the plane was up some steps and through a small door; Ian managed, appearing as nonchalant as he could. The floor inside was cushioned, so that was difficult, but then once in his seat he relaxed, after a fashion. His chair faced backwards and was in the middle of the plane, where g forces were studied best, to the right of the fuselage, with the other two experiments, an area for knee bending and the table to test reaching, in line across the plane. The others sat in forward-facing seats at the back. Ian noticed that there was no oxygen mask under his seat.[4] The zoot suit pockets were filled with small bags called "white carnations:" if someone felt sick they just pulled out a bag, vomited into it, tied it up, and then carried on.[5]

Ian well remembers taking off: "I was facing backwards, looking at 20 or so people seated at the back. With no windows and a plane taking off with a vengeance, I thought we were going straight up." Then they leveled off and got in position for the roller coaster. The plane was by now over the Gulf of Mexico and ready for four runs of ten parabolas. It would not stop unless someone was seriously hurt; vomiting did not count.

Jonathan sat at the table for the reaching task as the plane went over the top into zero gravity. The plane noise cut dramatically. Tethered to his seat, he felt his arm and body relax and loosen; a beautiful feeling, like swimming in clear warm water, only more so. He felt higher and longer, as his body stretched below his head and eyes, far more than before.[6] He knew that when he moved his arm would go too fast and too far but could not stop it. First time was bad, the second time better, and by the third time it was accurate; he had adapted to zero gravity. Then he looked down the fuselage. Everyone appeared to be on the ceiling. In zero gravity he saw the world as being upside down, even though when he looked down at his body that was still the right way up. These two seemingly impossible contradictions co-existed, and at no time during the transitions between gravity states was he aware of flipping back and forth between them; they just were.[7]

After 25 seconds, the pilot called out that they were bottoming out and 1.8g kicked in. The plane was shuddering as it went from 45 degrees down to 45 degrees up and was making a hell of a noise. Jonathan felt amazingly, dangerously, heavy and tense and knew his reach on the table would be too short and that his arm would bang into the table. As before, knowing that it would happen did not allow him to correct it until he had done it a couple of times.

After two sets of parabolas Jonathan moved to the knee bends. Standing up, the perceptions of zero and 1.8g were magnified. We have evolved in 1g and so are simply not aware of it. We feel no weight in our arms normally,[8] we do not feel twice as heavy if we stand on one leg or during the various phases of walking. The force of gravity is normally transparent. But, in 1.8g, if one stands on one leg it feels as if it's about to break under one's weight. Jonathan had to make a knee bend and then say how far down he felt he was, while his movements were recorded. In zero gravity he thought he had bent down far less than he actually did and, most curiously, as he bent down towards the floor, so the floor seemed to move away from him. He knew, intellectually, that this could not happen; he was, after all, bending his knees so his head and eyes had to be closer to the floor, but he still saw the opposite. In 1.8g, in contrast, he made small tentative knee bends, trying to avoid his legs breaking. He shouted out angles of big, deep bends as he actually made tiny dips ... and, as he made a small knee bend, the floor rushed up to meet him dramatically, the opposite of the effect in zero gravity.

After 38 of the 40 parabolas Jonathan had finished and just stood there for the last two, feet tethered, playing with the perceptions. He looked to the back of the plane and to the other experiments. There was frantic activity as everyone tried to finish. Further back, sitting on his own, was the legendary flight doctor Chuck La Pinta. Wearing a pink turtle-neck shirt, snakeskin boots, bandana, cowboy hat, and shades, and looking like a slightly bored understudy on *Apocalypse Now!*, he was calmly reading a newspaper.

Ian had not had such a good time. "I could have got a gold medal for vomiting. I puked for England; I soon gave up the slice of toast I'd had and then carried on retching on an empty stomach; the worst thing, I felt awful." Paul was amazingly adept at being there at the right time without being overly dramatic about it.

> My first test was with eyes closed. I remember as I went into the parabola and opened them there, in front of me 10 feet away was a Japanese guy in a ball in mid-air gently rolling around. Am I up, down, inside out, or what? I knew I was safe in my chair but there was no tug on the body. I had no idea which way up I was. I knew cognitively that I was strapped to the floor, but I did not know if that was down or up. By the rotating guy I knew it was zero g but I had no feedback from the arm or body. Nothing got into me to say I was floating or upside down. I had no clues and I had to fight an initial wave of panic. All those years of relearning the clues that enabled me to be safe, effectively accounted for nothing. Though physically safe strapped in, I was lost, drifting.

At 1.8g people feel amazingly heavy, but Ian remembers nothing of this. Despite feeling so ill, Ian did the experiments. However, at one point, unbeknownst to the others, his motion capture markers had become dislodged so his movement could not easily be reconstructed. The answer might have been more tape:

> The sensors coming loose really pissed me off, and it is not as if I hadn't pointed it out. A couple of dollars of tape negated all the work I and the team had put into this event. It raises a common issue; many researchers just don't listen to their subjects.

I put a great deal of time and effort into the projects I am invited to participate in, and I really do care about giving good results. Fortunately Jonathan didn't tell me for quite some time that my effort was wasted. He knows I would have exploded with anger and frustration.

NASA, being NASA, have a photographer on every flight. Jonathan had noticed that he was loitering around them and presumed it was because of Ian. But, once they had landed, the photographer explained that Marsha had told him to stick by Jonathan to take a photo of him being sick so she could e-mail it to his family back home. But Jonathan had not been sick, and so once on the tarmac he took Jonathan round the front of the plane to have his photo taken as a reward. Now, when a skinny physiologist is photographed in front of a plane at NASA in a zoot suit having just not been sick on the Vomit Comet, how should he stand? Shades on, he gave it his best Top Gun shot.[9]

Meanwhile, Ian remembers, while Jonathan was doing a photo shoot, he was still on the plane recovering:

> They were debating whether to take me to hospital while my guinea pig handler was outside having his photo taken. It was a good shot though . . . zoot suit, glasses, pose; pure Tom Cruise. . . . Wow what a flight, and certainly one that will stay in the memory. But no data successfully recorded. . . . I am gutted, and to this day I can't see a roll of micropore without feeling disappointed, and not a little angry.

They did offer Ian the chance of flying the next day. But, having been so ill the day before and concerned not to impose his disability on others, he declined. "Still, it was such an astounding experience; I would love to do it without the wires and the research and just go for the ride."

The next day Ian relaxed while Jonathan had 40 more parabolas, doing the sticks experiment with Jim, and also concentrating on the experience of zero and 1.8g. In zero gravity everything relaxed and though time was too precious to just float around, he was able to experience the sumptuous, voluptuous feeling of no gravity far better that the day before. Marsha said that on returning from a Shuttle mission she is homesick for space, and Jonathan could now understand that. In zero gravity even time itself seemed to relax and slow down.[10] As Jim said, gravity changes everything.

Perhaps the most interesting observation from the flight was that Ian had none of the illusions that most people have in altered gravitational fields:

> I never felt upside down, and I did not feel massive pressure under 1.8g. I had some pressure around the neck, but I really did not get a big disparity in perception between

reduced and increased gravity. I did not get the illusions; Jim Lackner asked me at the time and I did not.

He did not feel heavier in 1.8g, nor lighter in zero gravity. He did not feel upside down, he just lost all reference, and he did not get illusions of the floor becoming the ceiling. The feeling of heaviness and lightness felt by controls in different gravity conditions are so overwhelming that for Ian to feel nothing is itself extraordinary and, of course, suggests that these sensations arise largely through the nerve fibers he had lost.

Once disembarked on the second day we all trooped off to where Ian was waiting for a Cajun meal in a tin shack, famous as the place where astronauts have their final dinner before going down to Florida to fly. The food, Ian thought, was "Bloody awful." In contrast the shack was amazing with one wall covered with a photo of every astronaut. They settled down to eat under another wall covered in bumper stickers. Jim pointed one out, an advertisement for cigarettes. It read "Nine out of ten men who try Camels prefer women."

PERFECT DAY

Following his divorce Ian had moved back down south, wounded and poor. He found a place to live and bedded in with Stephen Duckworth's business. His attention to detail and commonsense approach soon gained him a reputation, and over the next few years he devoted himself to work and built up his savings.

One day, out of the blue, he had a phone call about website design for those with visual impairments. Brenda Coster, an information manager working for a consortium of probation services, had heard of Access Matters and wanted help. Over the next few months they phoned back and forth. Then, when she was in the area, they met over coffee. They got on well and she agreed to run some training courses for him. That was early summer; by that Christmas a strong friendship had developed.

Ian had never liked his house in Waterside and was looking hard for a new place. One day he was driving into the New Forest, a mile or so from his house, when he saw a chalet bungalow with a "For Sale" sign. He stopped the car and, taking the number from the sign outside, phoned the agent. It had only gone on the market that afternoon and the agent said he would find out if they would allow an immediate viewing. Ten minutes later the agent phoned back to say they would. Still sitting outside, Ian said he'd be with them in a couple of minutes. He looked round inside, liked it, found it was affordable, and phoned the agent with an offer. The owners accepted and took it off the market then and there.

That evening he phoned Brenda. "What are you doing for the weekend? Only I've just bought a house." Brenda came down and told him she thought it was nice but rather large. He replied that it wasn't just for him, he'd like her to move in with her two boys. That was the first she knew of it, and a few months later they moved in together. Her marriage was over and she was bringing up teenage boys on her own. She was a little surprised at how friendship turned so quickly into something else. Ian had no doubts:

> You would be lucky in life if you found just one person you totally fitted with. I have been exceptionally lucky; it has happened twice. With Brenda it all started innocently, and our friendship grew from there. I can't remember chatting much about

my disability. Clearly she knew about it by the time we met, but it wasn't a big topic, just something we got on with.

Brenda did find it curious coming to terms with Ian's condition and what he could and couldn't do:

> Once, we had gone to a garage for petrol and he asked me to fill the car up. He had asked this twice before, and so I said, "And why I am filling up and not you?" "I could do it but it would hurt my back and waste my energy." He never explained it properly, saying rather, "Read the book, or watch the *Horizon* program."

Brenda skimmed both; an in-depth understanding did not seem important:

> The strange thing was getting used to going to sleep with the lights on. I became more and more aware of what he was doing. A frightening time was when he had an ear infection. Until then I did not see how much of his cognition and vision and energy went into movement. With the pain he did not sleep for 3 days. By then he could hardly move. He'd go to grasp a cup off the table and miss it, his hand hunting and approaching it a number of times before pick up. For the first time I saw him mentally working out how to do things.[1] He always does that, of course, but you usually never see it.

Brenda went freelance with her business, working on systems analysis and data management within probation services round the country. Their new house in Rolleston Road was a new beginning for both of them. Brenda remembers going to the beach at Calshot to walk Daisy, her aging dog, with Ian sitting on the wall, throwing the dog her ball; a magical time watching ships come and go as they adjusted to each other's busy lives.

Felice, Ian's mother, was worried when she first came over from Jersey in case she did something in the kitchen that Brenda did not like. At that Brenda roared with laughter and just told Flossie, Ian's nickname for his mum, that she was not precious. "If she wanted to have a tea or make herself some food, whatever, just do it—it was more important for me she was relaxed." They all went out one Christmas morning to feed the ducks at a nearby pond and "to see the reindeer." As they walked back from a deer lookout, Flossie saw some glitter on the ground and was sad that a child had lost it. Brenda joked that it wasn't glitter but Santa's dust, used to get the deer to fly. There was a pause and Flossie burst out laughing, "I'm nearly 80, not 8." It was the start of a great relationship.

When walking on the Millennium Bridge for some filming [for Deborah Bull's *The Dancer's Body*], Ian phoned Brenda's dad who was a proud Londoner but had never crossed the bridge. The phone call meant a lot. He lived alone, and had recently collapsed. Once discharged from hospital he came down to Rolleston Road for recuperation. It was fluid on the lungs, caused by mesothelioma, and he needed repeated pleural taps; before long he died. Ian and Brenda looked after him as best they could at home. She remembers, "Suddenly Ian had two teenage boys wafting in and out, and a father-in-law dying . . . it was hard for him." She did not add how hard it was for her.[2] Ian remembers:

> To say the early months were tough doesn't go anywhere near explaining how chal-
> lenging it was. That we all survived says much about her strength of character. I loved
> her from the outset, but a new, deeper respect developed as I saw just how capable
> and courageous she really is. Brenda taught me a great deal about how to deal with
> adversity. I wouldn't want to repeat those months, but we are a stronger couple for it.

Ian worked at a frantic pace for several years. Disability Matters did well out of him and he was delighted to be earning so much, especially with so little formal training. Within a few months he had formed his own company, Access Matters, which subcontracted his services to Disability Matters. Then, after a while, he realized that he was only seeing a percentage of what Disability Matters charged for his services. He let it pass for a while but when he began to pick up some projects himself he asked Stephen Duckworth about the pay and whether he would make him a partner. Nothing came of it at the time.

Stephen was driven, firmly of the view that the best thing for people with im-pairments was for them to seek independence, where possible by working.[3] He had followed his own mantra and built up Disability Matters to employ over a dozen people and to function in several different areas: his consultant work and advice for companies, and increasingly for the government, on disability; his work as an expert witness in the courts in compensation claims; the training courses for newly disabled people and for companies and public bodies wanting to learn about dis-ability and employment; and, lastly, the physical access work which Ian and others had been so involved in. Stephen was earning good money from the first part, but began to find running the other parts of the business increasingly difficult. So he decided to move into the more lucrative expert witness work and separate this from the other parts of the company.[4] When he told Ian that he was going to split the company, Ian was shocked, thinking that his own income would be gone. But then, as he thought it through, he began to see an opportunity. The words of a few years earlier, that if they did not employ him he would be their main rival, came back to him. Might he take over the access part of the company?

He chatted to Mike, his immediate boss at Disability Matters. He had also thought of buying it but was not sure he could cope on his own. They decided to buy it to-gether, under Ian's company, Access Matters, and approached Stephen. He wanted to sell it for as much as he could, naturally; the problem was, as Ian pointed out, that without the Duckworth name it was worth nothing. After a short stand-off Ian and Mike bought it, for £1, the minimum amount for which a company could change hands. Mike and Ian became co-directors of their own company.

They had an office and some staff, a good cadre of clients and, with Mike's expertise in training and Ian's in access audit, all should have been well. Soon, however, it became clear that Stephen had managed Mike in a way Ian never could. The company had templates for audits, which Ian had helped develop and which were their currency and expertise. Mike, for some reason, gave several of these away to major companies. They had employed a freelance consultant to put together a web-based training package. Mike gave that away too. His expenses claims were also far too large. It did not help that, from the outset, Mike disliked Brenda intensely. He often downloaded non-work-related data onto their network, which had caused problems. Brenda, who was managing the Access Matters computer system software, knew it was him from her audit trails. Once, when Brenda asked Mike what he had downloaded, he went berserk, denying everything.

The company was set up with Ian's money, and while Mike drew a full wage from the outset, Ian didn't. Ian was working harder and harder to keep the business afloat as Mike was giving clients freebies. Mike was not bringing in much work either. After a year the relationship was untenable and Ian called Mike to a meeting one Sunday morning to tell him he was folding the company. Mike was incandescent, mainly about what people might say; for him it was all about "saving face." Eventually they agreed to split in an apparently amicable way. Ian was sad it had turned out that way; Mike had been a very good friend to him when he had first started to work for Stephen. But he had become a liability, in part because of his increasingly difficult behavior and in part perhaps because he never accepted Ian going from being his employee to his colleague.

Ian phoned all his own clients to tell them of the new arrangements. Several were relieved to be in Ian's hands alone. Ian kept his big clients—Intercontinental Hotels, Barclays TSB, Lloyds, Nationwide, NatWest Bank, the Post Office, RBS—and expanded his business as well. At one time Access Matters had 16 freelance consultants working on various projects around the UK. Although they had parted with an agreement that their respective businesses would be complementary, with Ian doing access work and Mike training, Ian found that Mike was undertaking access work too, so they were rivals. A few years later they heard that Mike had died suddenly at home.

Over the next few years Ian and Brenda built up their businesses, with Brenda doing more and more work for local authorities, especially on the Channel Islands, which meant short flights most weeks, while Ian's work took him to London and the north. He spent considerable time away on long trips cramming in as many clients as he could *en route*. He was working for John Lewis, a large and much respected retailer, for training events, for 100 Odeon Cinema premises, and a mobile phone network, Orange, with over 350 stores, among others. The money was good, but Ian was working all hours and was often on the road for days on end. By now he had closed his Stockbridge offices and worked from home. They both needed more space and Ian needed to be closer to a railway station. They started looking at houses again.

This time Brenda found the place. Wickham House was in the Meon Valley, just east of Winchester in a delightful semi-rural spot. It was a large double-fronted Victorian house, with a front drive round a sunken lawn and a thicket of trees and shrubs. Round the back were a double garage and some outbuildings. The house had huge, old windows with the original glass, and two verandas with wrought iron supports; one for the morning sun and another for the evening; beneath was a huge cellar. It was a big step up the housing ladder, though it needed lots of work inside and out. If the state of the house wasn't enough, there was another snag. The estate agent told them that a year or more before there had been a double murder in the house; a young man had killed his grandmother and aunt. The family had kept the house empty since then but now felt it time to move on. Neither Ian not Brenda was concerned, so they went ahead.

A couple of weeks after they moved in it was Ian's mother's eightieth birthday and she came over from the Channel Islands. She knew they were looking at houses, but didn't know they had bought one. They picked her up from the airport and said they had to look at a property on the way home. They took her to the house and went upstairs to the one decorated room in the house; her bedroom. They had put her slippers under the bed, and she saw them and said incredulously, "They are my slippers." "Yes," they said, "we have bought it;" she was delighted. Everyone who saw it loved it.

Brenda was spending more and more time on Jersey, and when she was there Ian would try to be at home. He would drop her at the airport and fend for himself quite happily for 1 or 2 days, working on audit reports. If he had an audit trip, Brenda would try to go too. Though he employed consultants, Ian, being Ian, was still very hands on. Like Stephen before him, he found it tiring and stressful to coordinate disparate people's work on various projects to ensure continuity in reports. Juggling people and maintaining standards became too much and they started talking about easing back a bit. Then Brenda fell.

One January evening she went out to the bins round the back of the house. It had snowed and, to avoid the slippery gravel track, she went over the fresh snow covering the lawn. Turning a corner, she slipped; her leg went backwards and she fell against a hedge in a drift of snow, snapping her leg just above the ankle. She cried out to Ian. "I've broken my leg," Ever sensitive, he replied, "Since when did you become a bloody doctor. Get off your arse and stop messing about." "I've broken my leg; call an ambulance?" "Are you sure?" "Well, I need an ambulance. I cannot move."

He rang 999 and gave the address. They said they would be there soon, adding, "Make the patient comfortable and keep her warm." The trouble was, in the dark and snow, there was no way Ian could go outdoors. He shouted, "I cannot get to you safely." "I am OK, just put the outside light on and keep talking to me."

The ambulance driver could not find the house and went straight past, three times. Ian phoned again. By the time they reached the house Brenda had been in the snow for 20 to 30 minutes. They immediately realized that it would take more than two people to lift her. So they covered her, gave her gas and air, and waited for the second ambulance, which in turn could not find them initially. Brenda lay on the snow for over an hour. The next thing she remembers is being in the ambulance, and the crew asking her to breathe and open her eyes. They thought they had lost her and were about to resuscitate, having stopped on the way to the hospital in a lay-by. She thought, "Oh, this is close." Once in hospital they warmed her frantically.

Ian did not go with her; he did not want to be responsible for another incident following behind and did not think he would be much help. Instead, he phoned her son Kevin and asked him to get to Winchester Hospital, fast. Only then did Ian set out, knowing Kevin could help him.

Brenda had a spiral fracture of the tibia and fibula and was in hospital for a week. Initially they were going to operate but then decided not to. A few weeks later surgery was required, though unfortunately the pins were not put in well and she remained in pain until several years later.[5] Ian managed with help from friends and family. Though Felice came over for a few weeks, the episode showed not only how vulnerable Ian was alone but also made them realize how hard they were working and how little time they had to themselves. They never took holidays,[6] and though they visited hotels it was never for leisure. Ian once worked out that they must have visited most towns in the England and all the motorway service stations. They had to do less. The difficult bit, as Stephen Duckworth had found, was finding a way to manage the process down.

They loved Wickham House, especially when filled with family. Ian had once said he missed kicking through the leaves, so one autumn Brenda picked up a bag full and then, when they sat out on the back porch, she emptied them on the ground at his feet to kick around. But, much as they loved the place, after 3 years they needed to downsize. Everyone thought they were mad to buy the house and now they thought them equally crazy to think of moving. But they could not sustain such a big property without a big business. They needed a more manageable place. They looked for something further west, smaller, and yet within easy distance of an airport for Brenda's increasing business in the Channel Islands. She looked for a bungalow; Ian for a house. She won. They found a delightful bungalow, Dodpen Farm, with 5 acres of land on the Dorset/Devon border just inland from the Jurassic Coast. Set at the top of a long valley, they could see for miles over fields and trees. Above them was a beautiful area of woodland, through which one has to drive to reach them down a narrow lane and then along a stone track. Brenda admits they bought with their hearts not their heads, but one can easily see why.

> Moving was the right thing, but moving here may not have been the most sensible way forward. We fell in love with the view, though living remotely down a potholed track, on the side of a hill, exposed to all elements of the weather, may not have been wise. But I absolutely love it.

Ian agrees:

> It is what I dreamed of as a kid, woods, wildlife, remote . . . a bit of paradise.

At Wickham Ian's brother had hacked away at the top of the garden one weekend and discovered a poultry house; old, dangerously rotten, and completely hidden by brambles. They decided that if the last people had kept chickens then so could they. Ian soon became passionate. "It was good fun looking after them and collecting the eggs. But, typical of me, I wanted old fashioned birds with brown and blue eggs like my grandfather had." Another piece of the jigsaw was their last Christmas at Wickham when Brenda had bought a traditional turkey from their local butcher. Though expensive, it was not a proper traditional bird either; it had never seen a field. Ian decided to explore sourcing a truly old-fashioned turkey for the following Christmas. He soon realized that there was a demand for rare breeds of turkey and decided to breed them once they were settled in the new place.

At Dodpen Farm a man was hired to bash in the fence posts, but they did the rest, Ian holding the posts as Brenda hammered in the nails for the netting. Within a few months they had gone from 4 small pens to 12 large permanent ones stocked with traditional varieties of turkey.

They travelled all over the UK for traditional birds with a good provenance. In Nottingham they sat-navved their way to a modest housing estate. Brenda knocked on the door of a small terraced house. The door opened and a woman emerged with two young turkey poults poking their heads out of her cleavage; she explained she was keeping them warm. They left with three gorgeous Bourbon Red turkeys. They took a 500-mile round trip to Manchester to pick up a trio of Narragansett turkeys. When they got there they discovered the hens were sitting on a clutch of 20 eggs. They decided to risk moving the hens and eggs and a week later 12 turkey poults had hatched.

At each house they have needed help and have been fortunate in finding the right people, excellent workers who are good fun. In Dorset, they needed someone to manage the poultry when Brenda was away and ended up with two people, one in the morning and another for the evening. It has worked out well, with flexibility for when Brenda was away, or if someone was away or ill.

Mike, the morning man, had been a teacher and taken early retirement and is reliable, punctual, and impervious to the weather. Fishy Pete, the evening man, is a wonderful, passionate figure and a natural stockman. A fanatical tea drinker, his passions include greyhounds, pugs, pigeons, pigs, canaries, parrots, koi carp, roses, fuchsias, hostas, irises, cross stitch, and ducks to name but a few, coupled with "off-beat" northern humor. He and Ian bonded immediately.

Brenda was well aware that with Ian's back problems and her work away he was very isolated should something go wrong. Mike and Fishy Pete were part of a safety blanket so there was always someone dropping in. Brenda has also been in touch with social services to see what is available in terms of help. Though Ian is reluctant to discuss this, Brenda has been quietly building up support. So much so that Dorset is the first area they have lived that she thinks they cannot leave, since they have a network for Ian:

> After much discussion I finally capitulated and asked the local authorities to help with a few adaptions. The turning point was falling in the bathroom and knocking out some teeth. It dented my pride, but I did the long interviews and endless form filling.

After all that he was refused:

> The real slap was being admonished for asking for help that wasn't actually meant for "people like me." Ironic, I have spent my life fighting for independence, now when I needed a bit of help it was to be denied. It's a funny old life at times . . .

With the recession Ian lost some contracts and found that the type of work changed. He becomes involved now when a client is challenged about access, or when there is a technical issue to resolve, rather than earlier and more routinely. Recently, though, he has secured a national project in the banking sector which will give him several years' work at his own pace. This is ideal, not least because he also has the birds to think about:

> It is not surprising I became more passionate about turkeys. After all I am a butcher and have always been passionate about local meat with a good provenance. It goes back to when I was in Jersey and going occasionally with Frank, my boss, to buy cows being "retired" from a dairy herd. Buying on the hoof you essentially got to see the process from start to finish, and then one certainly respects the carcass more. I always found it a humbling experience and am amused that the practical, honest approach to meat production from my youth has become "trendy."

They now have an increasingly well-known and respected flock of traditional varieties of turkey that mate naturally, rear their young competently, and are robust enough to range freely in all weathers. Truly traditional varieties—Bourbon Red, Bronze, Buff, Harvey Speckled, Narragansett, Pied, and Slate—Ian can reel them off with knowledge and pride. Their small-holding now has a dozen or so large pens with turkeys and a few chickens, geese, and peacocks, and was recently commended as being an ideal model breeding farm by the national organization. Their aim is to keep the traditional breeds going and to sell breeding pairs or poults on for others to rear for the table or, hopefully, to start breeding groups. They also have pigs occasionally, from which Ian had been known to make sausages, his butcher's skills re-awakened:

> I really love working with meat again, but it makes me realize the poverty of my situation and how much the disability has taken from me. Although I know all that needs to be done with the carcass it now takes such a time, and without touch, or the feedback from my knife, the old skills are diminished. I love the craft skill and get immense satisfaction from taking part in all stages of the process from field to table.

At the end of the season, they let each hen keep its final clutch. Then Ian can see how good they are at parenting—they do not breed from poor ones next season. In contrast, commercial breeds are usually artificially inseminated and never rear their own young, so one never knows how good they are as parents.

When Ian started he had nowhere to hatch the eggs, so he used artificial incubators, either in the spare room or kitchen. Sitting in the kitchen one was surrounded by several hundred chirping chicks, separated into the day olds, two-day olds, etc. In the corner of the room, every few minutes, a mechanical incubator would automatically whir into action and turn the eggs. Ian seemed oblivious to the noise; unsurprisingly Brenda was less keen and soon stopped it. After that the eggs were hatched in a large purpose-built wooden shed:

As long as the turkey project washed its face financially we would have been happy, but with the recession it now needs to provide an income. Every year demand exceeds supply, which is a great position to be in, so now it's just a case of ramping up what we do without incurring excessive labor costs. We like a challenge.

As the fame of their company, Heritage Turkeys, has spread, so they have received some interesting requests. One was from the catering manager for Kensington and Buckingham Palaces wanting turkey eggs as part of a demonstration of local produce. Ian promptly sent a dozen turkey eggs to each palace. His first thought on receiving an e-mail from a Native American Indian Chief, Billy Two Clouds, was that it was a wind-up. But it was genuine; Billy wanted turkey feathers to make a headdress. An eccentric titled lady bought a turkey as a companion; next week she sent Ian a photo of the turkey on her bed. They often get phone calls from people across the world, from Slovakia, Bulgaria, or South Africa, assuming they are a large commercial company and wanting anything from six to 10,000 turkey eggs. Although Heritage Turkeys cannot do large numbers they have sent eggs within the European Union to Italy, France, and Spain.

He has always kept a photographic record of the turkeys. About 2 years ago he had a phone call from a journalist who wanted pictures for an article. Ian asked who was writing it and she said, "Me." Ian said she did not seem to know much about turkeys; would she like him to write it? Without hesitation she replied, "Can I have it by Friday?" Thus Ian's latest career was born. He now writes regularly for *Grow Your Own* magazine on the management of turkeys. He has just finished a series for *Smallholder* magazine on how to rear turkeys "from hatch to dispatch," and is planning a book on managing turkeys. He has already written one book about disability access, with pre-publication orders of over 500. But, he says, turkeys are more fun, and the legislative implications less onerous. His reputation continues to grow, and recently he was voted onto the committee of the UK Turkey Club. Nonchalant when talking of this, underneath Ian was delighted.

Just behind the 16 miles of Chesil Beach, hidden in the steep, wooded Dorset hills, lies Abbotsbury Subtropical Gardens. There are 30 acres of mature trees and shrubs, with lakes and streams, a restaurant in an American-style Colonial Plantation bungalow and, set in a corner of the gardens, a small wooden "temple" licensed for weddings.

June 8, 2013 was sunny, clear, and bright. Ian arrived in suit and tie, and soon met up with his brothers, who looked slightly sinister in grey suits and dark glasses. Ian, taking Herb Schaumburg's advice, had bought an electric wheelchair. It had two speeds; full steam ahead and stop, a bit like Ian himself. Brenda had insisted that if Ian was sitting then so would she, and a wooden bench was arranged. The registrar managed just the right amount of solemnity and lightness, and within a few minutes Brenda's son Peter had given a reading and they had made their promises. They were married.

The speeches were short. Brenda's brother wondered aloud what everyone had been thinking, "Why had it taken Ian so long to propose?" Ian's elder brother, Colin, gave a short speech of appreciation while Ian managed to be witty, wise, and moving in his appreciation of his new family and of all his friends and relations for making it such a memorable day. He went out of his way to thank and praise his two new stepsons, his first family. Brenda's eldest son, Kevin, gave a speech appreciating that he could now officially call Ian "dad," declaring that to call him "my mum's boyfriend" never felt right. The best man related a few anecdotes about travelling abroad with Ian on research trips. At the end of the evening Ian and Brenda's estate car was filled with the left-over flowers. Kevin said it looked like a hearse.

Seeing a young couple committing their lives to each other is always touching. They have little idea what it entails but are ready for the challenge. Yet to see an older couple do the same thing, after previous marriages, hiccups, and setbacks, is often more moving. Seeing Ian and Brenda's happiness in each other, and them sealing it on such a perfect day, was a simple yet profound joy. Then they drove home to check the turkeys.

THROWAWAYS

Gesture in Chicago

When they were in Quebec together for a week of experiments Ian and Ginette had had little time to talk. Compounding this, she—being Québécois—spoke no English, while Ian—being English—spoke no French. They were filmed chatting once, with Michelle Fleury translating. Jonathan remembers little of what was said, and instead just sat watching Ian and Ginette as they conversed.

Ian sat with his hands resting on his lap. Just before he began to speak he glanced down and picked them up. Then, once they were before him, he spoke and gestured freely. As Michelle started her translation, Ian glanced down and parked his hands once more on his lap. Ginette was similar; she gestured as she spoke and then, when listening, rested her hands on her knees. Ian's gesture appeared fluent and free, especially since he was sitting down, but its take-off and landing needed visual supervision. In contrast, Ginette's was shakier, more ataxic, though equally expressive.

In *Pride and a Daily Marathon* Ian's gestures were mentioned—though only just:

> . . . sometimes I use [gesture], but only when sitting down, which allows me to do it without fear of falling, and I always have to think about it. I have to decide consciously to use my hands to move with and emphasize my speech.

Jonathan had written that though Ian seemed to move his arms and hands fluently, on closer inspection the fingers moved less expressively:

> Ian is always caught in a trap. Isn't thinking about movement the same as acting? And doesn't acting suggest artifice and untruthfulness? Ian has . . . regained some appearance of spontaneity, to communicate and conceal his actions, and hence his thoughts, by body language. [This] reacquisition depends on concealment that these gestures are in his case heartfelt but consciously made.[1]

That was nearly 25 years ago and since then Ian's gesture has undoubtedly improved in range and facility, and as we have visited labs it has attracted a lot of interest. In

Munich, Albrecht Struppler, a professor of neurology, had commented that he did not think Ian's gesture could be voluntary, seeing how skillful he was.

For his part Ian had not thought much about it, but this changed when David McNeill from the University of Chicago was alerted to his case by Shaun Gallagher, a philosopher and phenomenologist. David, emeritus professor of psychology and linguistics and a seminal figure in the scientific study of gesture, was immediately keen to study Ian.[2] We travelled to Chicago to meet David and Shaun, who had been lured towards the dark side of empirical work. David has described how he entered the field, his "language–gesture epiphany:"

> [At] a conference in Paris, at the end of 1971 . . . held in a lecture hall, originally set up for a diplomatic meetings, with translators at the back, overlooking the hall through a glass window from a soundproof booth, I noticed as I spoke (not then on gesture), a sight that at first baffled me. I could see a young woman behind the glass vigorously moving her arms in an alarming way. She looked to be having some kind of fit . . . until it dawned on me that she was translating me into French! The process of going from one language to the other, or just speaking itself, stimulated these movements of the arms. I believe I saw then, in a sudden apprehension via this distant yet strangely intimate connection of my speech to another person's movements, that language and gesture were two sides of one "thing." I can date my revelation this precisely . . . in mid-sentence.[3]

Ian, used to the eccentric interests of neuroscientists, was still surprised to learn of David's invitation:

> The thought that anyone would study my gesture was obscure. I had gone through my journey with it, in isolation. I never talked about it and no one had asked before. I did not think it a threat; in many ways I was quite interested.

Ian and Jonathan travelled to Chicago as part of the filming for the BBC's *Horizon* program and went over before the crew to acclimatize. Ian's back was painful at the time and, concerned not to exacerbate it, asked the BBC if he could fly business class. Without Ian there was no show, so they agreed—for him; Jonathan went tourist class at the back. Now Ian is last on a plane and last off, to avoid the jostling. He told Jonathan he would wait in his seat until everyone else had disembarked at Chicago. So, by the time Jonathan went forward to join him in business class, the cabin was empty. When a stewardess asked him why he was waiting, Ian replied, "For my doctor, he is travelling tourist class."

David had arranged for them to stay not far from the university in a motel on the North Drive. Jonathan's ground floor room appeared to be below a sort of gym. Occasionally there would be rhythmic sounds from the upstairs bed and then, soon after, a man would rush downstairs and disappear into the night. The TV crew turned up and heard there had been a murder at the motel recently. David was un-impressed; 2 years ago, he said, a plane had crashed onto the place.

Since his epiphany David had refined his study of gesture in immense detail using a deceptively simple technique. Following a previous researcher, Kendon, David distinguishes four types of movement with speech. "Gesticulation," is movement adding to meaning within speech, usually involving the arms and hands, though it may also be seen with the head and shoulders. "Speech-linked gestures" are parts of sentences themselves, or might complete a sentence (for instance we might say someone is in deep trouble by pretending to slit our throats). "Emblems" are con-ventionalized signs like thumbs up, while "pantomime" is a "dumb show," mime, a gesture or sequence of gestures without speech. David's interest is primarily in gesticulation.

David asks subjects to watch a cartoon starring Sylvester the Cat and Tweety, and then to retell the story while being recorded on video. Their gestures are then analysed in minute detail. He codes gesture in terms of parts—iconic, beat, metaphoric, and deictic gestures. An iconic gesture has a close relationship to the meaning of the speech, for instance if Tweety is going up inside a drain pipe, the gesture will involve the hand rising. Beats do not present meaning but are small rapid, rhythmic movements of the fingers or hands which seem to delineate timing of speech and gesture. But, as David told me, it also has deeper functions, a bit like yellow highlighter—emphasizing something in speech for its importance in a con-text beyond speech itself. So it is not just tied to the moment of speaking but reaches out to the larger framework. Metaphoric gestures also present imagery, but image as an abstract concept, such as knowledge or context, and often have two parts. In a question, one hand, the base, may be cupped while the other moves in an iconic gesture. Deictic gestures are pointing movements whether with finger or chin.

Movements are easy to see but very difficult to describe or analyze. David ana-lyzes gestures further in terms of the hands (handedness, shape of the hand, palm and finger orientation), motion (shape, direction), and meaning for hand, motion, and body. He also considers gesture space, a shallow disk in front of the speaker.[4] When describing something, the subject can also adopt his or her own perspective in gesture space, or that of a character being described, the observer or character viewpoint. And all this analysis is done in relation to the language being expressed, in terms of words, prosody etc., and frame by frame, millisecond by millisecond.

Science is best done methodically and quietly. At David's lab they had 2 days for introductions, experiments, and filming (including the BBC filming David film-ing Ian). David and his team's forward planning and the crew's sensitivity were a great help.

Ian watched the cartoons and then retold them under two conditions. In the first he could see his arms as usual. Then, in the second, David and his crew fixed a screen which sat in front of Ian so he could not see his hands, arms and body even though he could see the room. He repeated the performance, trying to gesture without visual feedback. They also filmed him chatting, with and without him being able to seeing his hands. Everyone was aware, most of all Ian, that they were trying to capture gesture when he was unaware of being watched, though this was difficult with cameras around and because Ian is so acutely aware of everything around him:

> I remember the Sylvester and Tweety Pie cartoon and then related it in a chair with the cameras on. You immediately perform; you don't lie but you do perform. I did it once with vision and then without, with a board between me and my body. I was aware that I should not make myself look stupid by doing exaggerated gestures. I sat comfortably and safely and gestured, for me, normally. I was trying to remember the story and recount it. I was not thinking of timings, I was doing it normally for me at the time. I was very aware of not forgetting the story and looking stupid, always conscious of the story. The gesture was as normal as it could be. I was not trying to outwit David or change anything normal for me.

Ian disliked cartoons and was also ambivalent about David's method. Ian felt David was like an anthropologist studying him at a distance rather than just spending some time being with him. Gesture involved conversation, between people, with turn taking and give and take; interpersonal interaction. Here, Ian felt, he was being asked to gesture on his own, in front of people he knew were studying him:

> Going to McNeill's lab, I had to say the bowling ball [in the cartoon] was on top, or dropped down. I can remember sitting there and thinking top/bottom, and putting it all together and thinking it all through, including what I was going to gesture before I did. But it is so unreal looking at gesture in relation to something, the cartoon, which does not mean much to me. It would have been better to have met him outside a lab and have a meal just chatting, and then he may have seen me differently. He had been watching people do the same task with similar gestures for 20 years, and I know I have to perform and then this [my] performance gets in the way.
>
> There were things about gesture that fascinated me; I was frustrated meeting him because he seemed to have a preconceived idea about his theory. I just did not think we hit it off. If we had chatted over a meal outside the lab, then he may have understood me a bit more and I would have understood him more.

To be fair to David he was trying to run important experiments while himself being filmed and under time pressure. (David, Jonathan, and Shaun did manage to acquire good data during the short time in Chicago with the BBC team, but also managed a second more leisurely trip a few years later, courtesy of Wellcome Trust.) David also needed to analyze Ian in his lab doing a similar task to others so he could compare Ian's performance in a controlled manner. Lastly, Jonathan always tried to avoid discussing the experiments too much with Ian, because as soon as Ian understands the aim his performance can change. This may have happened here somewhat, because David was not initially clear about Ian's resourcefulness:

> I wish he had not talked about timing of gesture, since then I started to think about it and I was no longer naïve to his purpose. You are stuck in a position in a lab with McNeill, having flown to Chicago, not for the parrots in the park, but for gesture. I wanted to do it as much with eyes shut as with open. I was trying to be as normal as possible and not over perform. There was always going to be less gesture without vision because I cannot see my hands. I was frustrated. I was still making movements but I felt the simpler ones were better, more secure. "He picked up a ball . . . Top of the drain pipe and then let go." I could do that stuff. But if I was having a complex thought then I cannot choreograph a sentence and gesture without vision.

He remembers the time under the screen very well:

> As soon as I cannot see my hands I lose contact with them. The saving grace was that before this I had to start thinking about where my hands were. I know how to make a square or a circle or a wave. I can do all these with vision and pretty well without vision. I tried cheating by looking in the camera lens, but there was no visual feedback. I knew my arms would drift. I still wanted to gesture and think I did the gestures but my accuracy went. I think he was surprised I did them as well as I did.

One of the first people to analyse language, and its relation to thought, was the Russian neuropsychologist Lev Vygotsky:

> Thought, unlike language, does not consist of separate units. When I wish to communicate the thought that today I saw a barefoot boy in a blue shirt running down the street, I do not see each item separately: the boy, the shirt, its blue colour, his running, the absence of shoes. I conceive of this in one thought, but I put it into separate words . . . . In [the] mind the whole thought is present at once, but in speech it has to be developed successively . . . the transition from thought to word leads through meaning.[5]

David has extended this to make a bold and original observation, that the unfolding of thought and language takes place coupled together in—and by—the unfolding of gesture. Language, it is suggested, did not evolve logically and cognitively but in the flow of life and in the rich soup of social interaction. Speech, of itself, seems incomplete without gesture; David maintains that the two co-evolved and, indeed, are mutually dependent:

> Language is inseparable from imagery and the imagery in question is embodied in the gestures that universally and automatically occur with speech. Speech and gesture

occupy the same time slices when they share meanings and have the same relationships in context. It is profoundly an error to think of gesture as a code or "body language," separate from spoken language . . . gestures are part of language. It makes no more sense to treat gestures in isolation from speech that to read a book by looking only at the "g's."[6]

It may need a deep breath to consider a gesture as imagery in this sense, but David's idea is that there are parallel meanings at play as we converse; language (words, phrasing, prosody, volume, and mood) and gesture. One unfolds in discrete packets of information, words and phrases, while the other proceeds at the same time but in a parallel series of longer movements. David's suggestion is that these two share and extend meaning between them and interact, with gesture facilitating and binding language in and through time. Language is more than words, it is social performance (so much so that we even gesture when speaking on the phone). Gesture shows how important it is for language to be embodied, to unfurl not only in speech acts, but in communicative acts within the body which complement the words and prosody of speech.

David's other suggestion is no less challenging—that gesture, "*the actual motion of the gesture itself*, is a dimension of meaning . . . gesture is the very image; not an 'expression' or 'representation' of it, but is it." Gestures and speech are then are not only "messages" or communications, but are ways of cognitively existing, of cognitively being, at the moment of speaking . . . .[7]

This follows Vygotsky's idea of a material carrier, an embodiment of meaning in a concrete enactment or material experience:

> By performing a gesture, a core idea is brought into concrete existence and becomes part of the speaker's existence at that moment. A gesture is not a representation, or it is not only such; it is a form of being . . . Gestures (and words as well) are themselves thinking in one of its many forms—not only expressions of thought, but thought itself. Meaning is never dissociated from the body; indeed it is impossible ("unthinkable") without engagement of the body.[7]

In his 2015 book, David challenges us to think of gesture and language as being inseparable parts of one whole and, in turn, to see them as performance, in real time, between people.

This may be fascinating, but where did Ian fit in? David suggests that there is a thought–language–gesture system, with the parts coexisting and co-dependent. In his second book, he develops the theory and suggests areas of the brain that might be involved in gesture: Broca's area and the area next to it, a mirror neuron area. Gesture, after all, has meaning for others as for us. If David were able to find someone in whom gesture is preserved when other types of movement—instrumental (dressing, writing, feeding, etc.) and locomotion—were degraded or difficult, then this would offer some support for his theory. Step forward the butcher from Jersey.

In his two visits to Chicago in 1997 and 2002 Ian was filmed gesturing with and without vision, and also doing simple instrumental actions, putting the cap on a flask, passing a silk through a napkin ring, with and without vision, to see if we could show preservation of gesture when other actions were degraded.

Minute observation of Ian's gesture with vision revealed that the movements were smaller than those of controls (for reasons of safety), fewer in number, and tended to be performed one by one. The only clue that control was unusual was that he tended to look down at his hands during some phases of gesture. But in terms of timing, and character and observer viewpoint, they were indistinguishable from normal.[8]

When the blind was placed in front of Ian, so he could see the room but not down to his body and arms, he initially did not gesture. He was scared he might fall off the chair; as he relaxed so gestures appeared. He remarked at the time that:

> I can see gestures in my head, but I am not sure if they are happening. The reason I am staring at a small patch on the wall is to try to visualize what my hands are doing.

He was able to make gestures, and their shape and timing was preserved. But accuracy in external positions in space was degraded. With vision he relayed the cartoon using both observer and character viewpoints, but without vision the latter was lost. However, it was clear that even without vision Ian could modulate the speed of gestures and speech in tandem, slowing them down and speeding them up together. Timing and shape were preserved even when he did not know exactly where his arms and hands were. As expected, without vision, he could not manage the instrumental actions David had devised (putting the cap on a flask, pulling a scarf through a napkin ring like a magician).

At one point Ian started to gesture and then, only several seconds later, did he remark that he was gesturing, as though he had become aware of this after the event. This might be more evidence in favor a link between language and gesture. Here Ian disagrees:

> No. I was attending to those gestures before I told him; I knew about them. Let me go over it again, it has intrigued me. My hands are under the board, I cannot see them and then he asked me to relate the story. I start and I am beginning to gesture and then I have already done some before I say I am gesturing ... I would be aware I was doing them. I would never not be aware, because I would be aware of telling my hands and arms to do something. Since I was doing it, I would be telling them what to do.

I would be aware of initiating and of making the command to make it, and so assume it had happened.

Still, a lot is made consciously; a wave or whatever is supervised. I need cognitive effort to make sure they were controlled with no wide sweep. Sitting here, in a chair, if I were to get angry I would still have to be aware of my limits.

There is a hierarchy of control. Ian may not be aware of a gesture itself, but he has to be aware of how large and far it is and how it might change his center of gravity, and its consequences. Ian has a kitten, and recently it clawed him playfully. Ian made a sweeping movement to stop her, more intent on reaching his target than being safe; he nearly fell out of the chair:

It was refreshing to move without too much thought, but I realized I had to be more careful and controlled. I was not thinking about the implication of movement but its goal. Now, back in language and gesture, if I get swept up in long sweeping gestures I am aware I could fall out of the chair. I had to learn where and how far to gesture.

Ian rarely wants to know about the experiments he has taken part in and he does not always remember much about them. But he was interested in these gesture experiments, so Jonathan showed him various parts of the most expansive papers and books that David has written on him. In one paper David and his team consider the way in which gesture and speech interact in a way that, in turn, surprised Ian:

At one point in the 2002 experiment Jonathan Cole demonstrated, as IW watched, an object-directed transitive action [removing the cap from the flask]; IW then imitated the action.

While he could not perform the action himself without vision [as expected], we were interested in seeing if he could imitate it under conditions where topokinetic accuracy was not a factor, and indeed he could. But what was unexpected is that IW spontaneously spoke as he imitated the cap removal (he described his movements as he performed them). This was a fully spontaneous and unanticipated performance, not something we suggested, even though, of course, a spontaneous sprouting of speech is what our hypothesis implies—the two forms of materialization co-occurring.[9]

Ian had never thought of that and was really surprised that he had used language spontaneously to try to improve his movement—or to put it another way—that language had arrived, like the cavalry, to try to improve it. A parallel observation was made on another occasion:

The inverse experiment happened equally accidentally in a separate study of IW by Bennett Bertenthal (personal communication). Here, too, imitation was the task (he was shown a video, without sound, of other people's gestures and asked to imitate them). As before, IW spontaneously began to speak. The experimental assistant asked him to not speak, as that was not part of the experimental protocol. IW complied and—the important observation for material carrier purposes—his imitations immediately simplified and shrank dramatically in size. Whereas, with speech, they had been large, complex and executed in the space in front of his body (he was not under the blind), without it they were simple, miniaturized and confined to the space at his lap. This was so even though imitation of other people's gestures was his target and he had vision of his hands.

These effects are impressive indications that two materializations, speech and gesture, co-occur, support and feed one another, and that when one goes awry or missing the other tends to follow.[9]

Ian read this passage wide eyed. "That is interesting—fascinating—amazing. Being told to shut up and I gesture less! If you think about it, it ties in with gesture and language being together. That is neat." Jonathan explained that this is David's theory, that there is a thought–language–gesture system organized within the brain separate from the systems for other types of movement. Ian still sees another dimension. When gesture affects his safety or balance he has to control it appropriately and cognitively. "Sometimes the thought process regards gesture is really early on such as when standing, and at other times, with little or no safety implication, it flows more easily."

Jonathan continued that, when relating the cartoon, Ian had taken both the observer and the character viewpoints with his eyes open, but that without vision his use of the character viewpoint reduced. Without vision he retained his own perspective, of course, but could not represent that of someone else. Again Ian was surprised, not least that with vision he did both in the first place:

I can understand why it would be diminished without vision. I am just constructing safe, simplified gestures. With vision I can be more playful. I was not aware that I would take another perspective. Fascinating.

The paper continued to its final conclusion:

To end this section we will apply phenomenological philosophy to understand better the distinction between IW's "throw-aways" and his "constructeds." Recall that his constructeds were fewer in number, were isolated, performed one-by-one and in a self-conscious manner.

On the other hand, he produces his throw-aways with ease, though with some topokinetic problems. In a sense, by making this distinction, IW summarizes the whole point about the impossibility for third-person empirical-scientific approaches to fully capture the nature of gesture.

When IW is unaware of his perfectly synchronized gesturing (when he is producing what he calls "throw-aways"), he is immersed in the participatory point of view and he engages his whole body-as-subject to convey his intentions. He body enacts his cognitive being at that time. However, when he is constructing his constructeds, he takes an observational, detached and external stance towards his own performance. He consciously divides up his utterances and hand movements by objectifying their features and then tries to attain synchrony. He takes a meta-cognitive stance (trying to control his hand movements) which clashes with and disrupts what he is trying to express with his hands (whatever the conversation is about). Co-expressiveness of gesture and speech breaks down—and so does synchrony, and to some degree so does the sense-making process.[9]

Long words but, once more, Ian agreed. He knows that when gesturing from a secure posture and with an uncluttered gesture space he can go with the flow and that these are his most automatic movements. But he also knows that he has to think about some more complicated gestures, and despite his best intentions the flow of speech/gesture is then discontinued and fractured. Why then should he bother to make these designer gestures?

Part of the answer may be because, despite David's analysis, Ian is still not convinced his gestures are normal. He finds that in some details, not maybe in timing or shape but in the finer use of his fingers and hands, he is relatively impoverished. He cannot use fingers individually and so he tends to hang the fingers out during gesture, with broader flexion/extension of them rather than the more eloquent and articulate finger coordination used by others. Ian tries to refine gesture to appear more "normal" and arguably more eloquent, but he has to use cognitive effort for this, and sacrifice flow for effect. The other reason is simpler. He has a "hit parade" of gestures and quite likes thinking new ones up and trying them out. But this is dangerous ground for him, in relation to expression and manipulation of expression, albeit for the best of reasons:

> Talking about gesture is such a nightmare. I don't live in another world; it is the same one as everyone else and I have done so much to make me look the same. I have done so much which is a façade . . . I was worried I put up a charade and then spontaneity is out the window. I did not want to be seen as an actor.

People have been intrigued: if gesture and language are so linked, because Ian has to think to an extent about both, then which comes first?

> Don't ask me. I do actually think about things before I say them. And think not only about what I say but how I gesture it as well . . . I could not differentiate whether it was the movement or the gesture or the word I was hunting for. I gesture for me and for you. You cannot differentiate.[10]

David's analysis suggests that, in timing and in relation to spoken language, Ian's gestures are normal, supporting his theory of gesture being part of a common gesture and language system within the brain related to thought and communication, and separate from other areas to do with the movements of walking or, say, dressing. But Ian still has some misgivings:

> I don't think my gestures are normal, though some tics and shoulder shrugs are close .... The shape of my gestures and use of my fingers is less; it is too difficult. If someone was sad enough to analyze it then they would see that I do less precise finger stuff. I also think I gesture more than most.

There is one aspect of gesture other than timing and shape that should be considered. Jacques Paillard, who studied Ginette many times, made a distinction between topokinetic and morphokinetic movements.[11] The former have to be accurate in relation to place either in the external world or within the body (egocentric) space. For Ian to pick up a glass, for instance, he has to control the movement of his arm and hand to a precise point and then grasp and lift. In contrast, morphokinetic movements are those in which the shape of the movement is critical but its position in space is not. One might think of a classical conductor's use of a baton. But the most morphokinetic movements of all are gestures, which have form and shape but are not—crucially—accurate in place. Ian volunteers that morphokinetic movements are far easier. He loves driving a car, using a hand control for acceleration and braking and monitoring steering as much from what happens outside the car as from moving the steering wheel (like everyone else). Most of these movements are relatively easy and relaxed for him. He prefers driving 300 miles to filling the car with petrol, with its standing and manipulations of petrol cap, nozzle, and the payment; all complex mainly topokinetic movements.

The question, therefore, is whether gestures are easier because they lack the need for accuracy in place (though not time) or whether it is because their control is through a different system. Shaun Gallagher has written of a middle position, which he calls an "integrative theory of gesture."[12] In this he suggests that the initiation and timing of gesture is normally tied to communication, non-consciously, as David suggests, as is the morphokinetic shape of gestures, but that the topokinetic component, if there is one, cannot escape from the usual requirements for accurate movement, namely proprioceptive feedback, to allow the brain's motor apparatus to control movement. Such a model would allow Ian's gestures to be shaped and timed similarly to other people's but that their positional accuracy, in the absence of proprioception, depended on vision and thought.

Where Ian would disagree is over the initiation of gesture, for which he thinks he retains awareness, and in his rather more complex hierarchy of control, where he has to monitor his own safety and set the limits to gestural movement consciously.

But though Ian took some convincing about David's theory, he has much sympathy for it, especially after he understood the sophistication of the analysis, which, for once, out-reached his own analysis of what he was doing.

There are two other observations in favor of David's theory. As Ian suggests, he does gestures more than most people. But he also gestures in long streams of action, as we all do, in a way very different from his other actions. If he walks along a street, he will stop after 10 or 20 yards or so to relax slightly and to plot his next moves, like a climber going up a pitch. Similarly, when he eats or writes he pauses every so often. His actions are discontinuous and limited in time, as he thinks and plans and relaxes. In contrast he gestures continuously, for far longer and more naturally, without the need for pause or planning.

Another question is whether Ian was deprived of gesture by his illness and then had to relearn it or whether it continued, albeit in a slightly haphazard and uncontrolled way. Clues come from the first days and weeks after the neuronopathy:

> I don't think I ever lost gesture; I was never totally like a puppet without the strings, it was never gone completely. What happened was that I had less opportunity to manage it. I don't think I ever stopped gesturing completely. I remember clouting my mum round the ear with my hand during a gesture because I had not controlled it. In early days I had to think about my arms. Chatting away I would move my hands and have a problem. I certainly knew early on that communication was different.

Rather, he learned to reduce gesture until he found a way of managing it. Just as the first time he sat up he lost concentration and nearly fell out of bed, so the first time he made an expansive gesture, with his arms out to his side, he all but toppled over. Even now when sitting on an open stool or a bench he does not gesture, for safety's sake:

> To move round, to look behind me, I have to control movement, but to gesture I don't control it to anywhere like the same extent. The desire for movement with words was always there. It is how I am, how we all are.

Jonathan and Ian were once chatting away, with the former unaware of his own gesture:

> Even that gesture you made, with the arm sweeping up in front of you, would have had a problem for me. Scratching your forehead as you did then was OK because I could feel it on my head, but any precision gesture I think a lot more about. I just know the desire to make gesture was still there from the beginning; the switch or mechanism was always there. Gesture was unbidden, uncontrolled, unsafe, so

I supervised; I learned how far I could go. I learned quickly that if I pointed too far in one direction I would fall over. So I kept it in closer, honing it and looking. Now some gestures are automatic.

Most people with sensory loss are ataxic in their movements, their arms and fingers moving shakily. Ian initially found this too, when dressing or reaching for something. But he is less certain that his gestures were ever ataxic:

> Like Ginette, I 'hunted' in action, but not so much in gesture. If I tried to reach for a pencil, then I could not have done that in the early days. But in a gesture there is no end point, there is just a moving ellipse or gesture, and those were easy once you know how far you can go without toppling over. I don't think they were ever ataxic.[13]
>
> The impulse was always there, but I had to manage it more early on, and now I manage it less. Gestures wanted to be there so I had to manage them. Did I prune some? Yes, but I could not tell you what the fine line is between deciding to gesture and just doing it. Initially, remember, I was a wreck. But as soon as you became sociable again you gesture;[14] uncontrolled and without finesse . . . The gesture was there but to release it I had to be safe. I maybe did not need to think about the gesture I did, but I did need to think about being safe as a consequence of the gestural movement.

That gestures are normal in timing and synchronized with speech in Ian lends credence to David's theory. That they were never gone, wanting to be there "unbidden and uncontrolled," is surely further strong evidence. But Ian has to set their bounds to remain safe, initiates them, and has to supervise them visually; normally he would not gesture in poor light. Their spatial accuracy is also poor, when—rarely—this is required. In other words gesture may be related to thought, language, and communication but even Ian cannot ignore the fact that control of movement by the brain has limits without proprioceptive feedback.

Once, when chatting, Jonathan asked about the "tip of the tongue" phenomenon, making a gesture to bring out a half forgotten word. Ian found this works for him:

> It helps me to be more articulate in speech. . . . Not only more articulate in getting my message across but in helping me use language better. I can see my arm my moving and can feel it.

Feel it? He corrected himself:

> I can only see it and if my eyes are closed or I am in the dark I will not gesture. I got pleasure, in the early days, from learning to reconstruct gestures. I would congratulate myself on conversing pretty well, making gestures like letters in the alphabet. Sometimes I would be creating gestures consciously, even though there was always a willing inside wanting to do them. But something stopped me; I was putting myself in danger to do them. Some were denied and I could not be fluent because it was unsafe. But I do remember playing with some gestures I thought, and constructed,

and learned. If we had videoed it you would have seen them. I learned gestures, like I learned other movements and knew they were safe. Once learned, I just do them, unless I get carried away or I am doing them precisely. The willingness was always there and I knew initially that I was bereft of them.

If Ian's gestures include some of his most automatic movements, might he enjoy them? His answer was ambiguous:

I get pleasure after a conversation by getting by, in that people have not seen me as disabled. When I didn't gesture in the early days, to be safe, they noticed. It used to give me great pleasure to appear normal, but it's less so these days. But I do get fun from being successful in appearing normal and people not being aware of my problem.

You once asked me whether I just move or whether I act as I walk. I thought, "What a shit question." I started thinking, "Do I play with movement; do I play with gesture?" It is so difficult to pin down. It all began so long ago, I cannot remember. I wish we had met sooner after. What cannot be explained in words could have been explained visually. You'd have seen what began as a constructed cognitive movement switched into a simple throwaway . . . that would have been fascinating. Compared to walking, gestures are easy. All those bits I have to put together for walking; foot there, leg rigid, how balanced, wind, how fast, how safe? You cannot play when walking, I cannot play picking up a cup.

But it did seem he was able to gain some pleasure from the act as well as its effect on others:

I can be more flippant with gestures. Now I can do them more spontaneously they are more automatic and they are fun. Once I have set their boundaries, then I am off, and then I can play. In gestures I can relax into it. They now do it themselves, until the boundaries of wild sweeps, which topple me over, are reached.

He soon returned, though, to his original point:

I get some fun thinking I got away with it. It used to be an effort to do any; now some throwaways are as spontaneous as they can be. It's been a long journey and when I met David I was only half way there. Now I enjoy seeing my hands move, and making them move.

Once, I walked to end of the track where we live;[15] that was the greatest satisfaction I have ever had in movement since I acquired my disability. But the greatest spontaneous satisfaction is from gesture; because it is now like everyone else's again.

10

FEELING THE WARMTH

Touch Ian, stroke him, or put a heavy weight in his hand and he cannot feel it. For all the world he has no sense of light touch; nothing in daily living is felt on the skin unless it is hot, cold, itchy, or painful. It was therefore a surprise that Ian's threshold to von Frey filaments—carefully designed thin filaments which, when pressed on the skin, bend beyond a certain force—was near normal over his arm and chest. These filaments have always been thought to test the A-beta large sensory nerves that detect light touch, which Ian and Ginette lack over their bodies. But when we tested Ian's thresholds in the early 1990s they were just above normal, so we had to rethink.[1] We presumed that the monofilaments actually activated nerve endings conducting to the spinal cord and brain via the smaller C or perhaps A-delta fibers that are still intact in Ian, possibly because the ends of the filaments are sharp right angles and so are felt as "low-intensity" pain. Ian, in turn, had always said that he used pain and pre-pain when he could, though we were not entirely sure what pre-pain meant. Maybe the monofilaments were an example.

Peripheral nerves actually seem relatively simple. Sensory ones come in different shapes and sizes. The largest, A-beta fibers, are wrapped in a myelin sheath; they are the fastest and conduct impulses conveying touch and movement and position sense (at around 50 m/s). The next, A-delta, are smaller myelinated fibers involved in the perception of pain and temperature, while the smallest and slowest, C fibers, also underpin different aspects of pain and temperature. While A-deltas are involved in cold perception, C fibers convey perceptions of warmth. The differences in the pain conveyed may be illustrated by putting one's foot in a hot bath. There is an early sharp pain, thought to be from activation of A-delta fibers, and a later, delayed, pain which lingers and is unpleasant, the C fiber perception. A-deltas conduct at 12–14 m/s and C fibers at 0.5 m/s, so signals from C fibers reach the brain a second or so later.[2]

Ian has normal perception to pain and temperature, and is often asked if he finds he can use this perception for other things too, to help guide movement. Both Ginette and Ian use temperature to tell them if their hands have moved or their arms have drifted, but this does not allow them to know where they might have moved to. Vision is Ian's main replacement for proprioception:

> Vision is the biggest, by far, for safe mobility. But I also use sound, say someone walking up behind you. Waking up in bed in the morning, I will know my leg has moved by temperature clues. But I also know I can only get into a few positions during the night, so now it is easier.
>
> Pain is useful too; in standing and moving, I listen to twinges from my body. A bit of back pain makes me aware of leaning over too much, even in a wheelchair. I am now much more aware of the consequences of any action. I used to do this in immense detail and then I got cavalier; now I am back to being careful, with tensing, leaning over, and stretching. Pain tells me I have sat too long, or that I ought to stop doing something.

But none of these sensations is refined enough to guide movement; they are also too slow. C fibers may also be involved in the conduction of impulses elaborated into peripheral fatigue and cramp sensation from muscles, and these also appear to be normal in Ian. But since peripheral nerve function was first assessed, another type of C sensory fiber has been known to respond to light touch stimuli in a curious way, the function of which was uncertain. These low-threshold C fibers are found in hairy skin, but not over the smooth skin of the palm and sole of the foot, the so-called glabrous areas. In 1939 Yngve Zotterman suggested these might be involved in the perception of itch. As often happens, further insights into these fibers required a new technique.

In the 1960s and 1970s two Swedish physiologists, Åke Vallbo and Karl-Erik Hagbarth (with others), made small, fine needle electrodes which they pushed through their own skin directly into a peripheral nerve, say at the wrist, elbow, or knee.[3] They managed to record directly from nerve bundles. They were able to map the receptive fields of individual nerve cells and to characterize, for the first time, the types of sensory nerves and skin receptors in humans. Not only that; small currents could be passed through the electrodes to stimulate each nerve cell and the subjects asked what they felt. A single shock to a single A-beta axon could be felt, localized on the skin, and perceived according to the type of skin receptor the axon innervated. This work is astonishingly precise and demanding; it might take hours to position the electrode in the right place and then find a single nerve cell to record from. If the subject moves, or the experimenter coughs when moving the electrode, all could be lost.

The large A-beta nerve fibers were relatively accessible with these techniques. But even the far smaller C fibers began to be isolated too in the small groups or fascicles in which they lay and, with this, Zotterman's curious C fibers attracted interest once more. The cutaneous receptors of these nerve cells responded to slow weak stroking more than faster, strong strokes. Their response profiles to different speeds of stroke on the skin paralleled the perception of pleasantness felt during those strokes too, unlike the responses of the A-beta cells. These "CT" fibers may therefore underpin, say, the pleasant feeling of silk on the skin or a slow stroke across the arm, leg, or foot. They seemed to allow a link between nerve signals and emotional contexts; say the feel of a caress. In other words CT fibers might underpin social touch.[4]

A major problem was how to show the role of CT fibers in perception in humans, since any touch on the skin overwhelmingly activated A-beta fibers; selective activation of CT sensory fibers by stroking the skin was impossible in control subjects. The obvious ploy was to find someone with CT fibers but without A-beta fibers. Then one would not need to do micro-neurography but could just stroke the skin knowing that CT afferents would be activated in isolation. The problem was that neither Ginette nor Ian volunteered any sensation of touch whatsoever when touched, stroked, or caressed on the skin. What was needed was cunning.

This was provided by Håkan Olausson and colleagues studying Ginette in Montreal and Goteborg.[5] They showed that she could not feel light vibration (a pure A-beta stimulus) over the affected skin below her face but that her perceptions of cold, pain, and mild hot and cold pain were near normal. Then they used a small artist's brush and stroked her forearm. They asked if she could feel anything, and she was quite sure that she could not. But then they said, "OK, you cannot feel anything, but now you have to say if you were touched or not, even when unsure." Using this "two alternative forced choice" method she was able to say accurately whether she had been touched or not, much to her surprise.

Then they asked what it felt like, even though she was not quite sure what "it" was. If she concentrated hard, she said, she still had no perception of touch, but she could feel a faint diffuse sensation of pressure and volunteered it felt pleasant rather than painful, hot, cold, itchy, or tickly. Surprisingly, even though it felt far weaker than the feeling of the brush in controls, Ginette rated it equally as pleasant as they did. It appeared she had partially dissociated a feeling of touch from one of pleasure. She had however, no idea of whether the brush stroke was going up or down her arm.

Ginette was put in a brain scanner and her arm stroked. Control subjects in this situation activated the expected areas of the contralateral somatosensory cortex, S1 and S2, known to be where A-beta nerves projected, as well as the contralateral pre-motor cortex and parts of the insula cortex. In contrast, Ginette's responses were seen only in the insula areas, a little in the pre-motor cortex, and not at all in S1 or S2. Moreover, there were three areas on the insula with measurably increased blood flow, one that also receives heat pain and itch, one that also receives noxious and innocuous stimuli, and another that is also activated during romantic love and visual sexual arousal.

Here was evidence of what CT fibers might do. They might be nothing less than a parallel sensory system, separate from the light touch A-beta one both peripherally and in its connections in the brain. It responded to slow stroking touch, and so might be involved in "affective, emotional, hormonal and behavioural responses" to touch. This is crucial in mammals; rats fail to thrive if they are not licked and groomed by their mothers, while a newborn calf is licked and licked by its mother for hours. Non-human primates use gentle touch, grooming, as a way of social bonding. But such interpersonal, gentle, touch is also important in humans.[6]

In science more data are usually better; the obvious thing was to repeat and extend the experiments with Ian. Ian, Francis McGlone, a neuroscientist from Liverpool with expertise in this area, and Jonathan went to Goteborg.[7] Ian was quite claustrophobic and found the scanner environment difficult. Lying on the sled was also uncomfortable. The result, however, was the same; slow stroking led to activations in the insula areas and none in sensory cortex. Such a finding, in trying circumstances, reinforced just how secure and robust the result was. Not only were there activations in the insula areas but there were also de-activations of cortical activity in the sensory cortex, area S_1.[8] Reanalysis of Ginette's data, informed by data from Ian, showed widespread deactivations in her too, in contralateral S_1, bilateral S_2, and many other areas. When working, the CT system seemed to reduce processing in other sensory systems. In other words, when being stroked pleasantly one might feel other types of touch differently. Of course, although these sensory systems had been studied separately they would normally work together. Since activation of CT afferents does not lead to perception in most people, they may be working at a level below consciousness to instruct sensation from other pathways for contextualization (as will be elaborated later).

As with many experiments, especially those that don't require Ian to perform, he remembers little of this work. After all, when lying down and passive he does not need to remember. The problem was also that the feeling, if that was what it was, was so subtle Ian found it difficult to detect anything. Even when he was above chance levels when forced to respond, it was still too faint. "If all I am doing is attending to subtlety, then I could probably get it. But if it was that subtle in everyday life, I could not feel it. I don't remember what it felt like at all."

There was another problem, however, a deeper one; how to express such vague "almost perceptions." "I am frustrated; at times as a subject I am required to say what I feel and I cannot express it; there are not the words."

Jonathan mentioned that Ginette had volunteered that the faint brushing was pleasant. Ian was a little concerned by this:

> But if it's not unpleasant, it has to be pleasant. It goes back to language. If I concentrate hard and can feel something, then if it is not pain it has to be pleasant. It can only be either/or. If you feel it and it is not painful, nearly everything else is pleasure.

Subjects with reduced taste and smell have reported that when they do smell—anything—it is always pleasant, whether a woman's perfume, bacon sizzling, or sewage. Perhaps if you don't normally feel anything, then anything which is felt is perceived as pleasant. Ian agreed. "Yes there is something in that. Searching for a sensation, if it doesn't hurt then it is pleasure."[9]

There was one experiment in Goteborg with Ian in a MRI brain scanner that he did remember. He was stroked on the inside of the leg either by Brenda or by a Swedish nurse (who was introduced to Ian beforehand). The aim was to investigate the effect of context and relationship on brain activations to pleasant touch. The slight problem was that, if anything, Ian was more aroused (in functional MRI terms) by the Swedish woman.

If stimulation of CT afferents might be—at best—on the borders of perception, how do they usually function? After all it seems very unlikely that we feel CT-mediated touch when bombarded by the far more powerful A-beta system. Instead CT input may instruct the A-beta system to interpret a slow touch stimulus emotionally, as something pleasant. The great English physiologist Charles Scott Sherrington suggested in 1900 that, "Mind rarely, probably never, perceives any object with absolute indifference, that is without 'feeling.' All are linked closely to emotion."[10] Maybe the beginning of the perception is not only in "the mind" but in the neurophysiology of sensory perception at a pre-conscious level.

Some have suggested that the CT system works a little like blindsight. In this condition subjects with an area of blindness in their visual fields, due to a lesion in the visual cortex, can still respond to a visual stimulus in the blind area, even though they have no conscious awareness of it. Like Ginette and Ian, they deny awareness of a visual stimulus but, when forced to respond, they are better than chance at localizing or describing the object in their "blindsighted" visual field. But blindsight occurs with a cortical lesion, whereas here we are considering the normal role of CT afferents. Perhaps a better model may be photoreceptors in the mammalian retina which have been found to be involved not in vision but in synchronizing circadian rhythms with daylight.[11] These differ from the classical rod and cone (black and white, and color, respectively) photoreceptors in several ways, for instance in using a different photopigment, in having a lower sensitivity to light, and a lower spatiotemporal resolution. CT afferents may parallel these cells in not normally being felt. Whereas these retinal cells appear to control our day/night rhythms in relation to daylight, the CT afferents appear to work with the other main touch pathway, in A-beta fibers, to contextualize and tune our perception of, and emotional response to, touch.

Ian was interested, but said that these were not things he could play with or manipulate in any way. Neither could any of us, Jonathan replied, this all takes place below any conscious level. But the CT system did allow us to consider skin not just as an organ of touch, but an organ that is also enormously important for pleasurable touch in a variety of contexts, whether this is the brush of silk, the feeling of wind on the face, or within an intimate relationship.

CT afferents may be important in pleasant touch, but they are not the whole story. They are not present, for instance, on the palm of the hand, a crucial area of our bodies for affective or pleasant touch. We enjoy being caressed, but we also enjoy the act of caressing, though it is difficult to know whether our pleasure is from the hand or the context. Ian agrees.

> I still want to stroke the cat or run a hand over a nice object. When the cat comes in at night, damp, I will stroke her. I like the feel of wet.[12] I like to feel both animate creatures and inanimate objects. With a cat you want to engage and sometimes you feel it warm, or damp-cold. I still want to run my hand over the curve of a vase, even though I get nothing from it. I have no explanation for that and no feedback. I just get closer to it by moving my hand over it.

He might retain a faint memory of what it felt like to run his fingers over something, or he might have some equally faint percept associated with making the movement in his head, or he may gain some satisfaction from seeing the movement and touch unfold.[13]

Ian was clear that, despite his lack of cutaneous touch, tactile intimacy remained important, though differently. "When you put your arm round someone, you join with someone, there is relationship; you feel the warmth." How cruel then that, despite this, even when being intimate, Ian has to think about and be very careful how he moves. He cannot surrender to the moment completely.

> You learn to set limits. In the early days it was quite interesting. I had to learn boundaries, and be less adventurous; no more swinging from chandeliers. If I hug someone close it is no different to picking up a heavy object in terms of the physics

of movement. How far can I reach? How do I balance? I had to explore the physical side and that's why you need an understanding partner, leaving aside the problems of geometry and falling out of bed, which I did a few times. I have always loved textures, silk or rough; but these are not tactile any more. I used to get turned on by silk. Now there is nothing but a memory. It is not about the feedback, I have the memory and the moment. But for flesh against flesh it is different . . . and temperature plays its part. . . .

Ian was young when he became ill, and even though his sense of touch was gone, he remained otherwise intact, even early on in the Wessex Neurological Centre:

You cannot be a young man and have attractive young nurses bending over you doing intimate care without something stirring. I had an erection at times during a bed bath, though I would try to think of something else. There were embarrassing moments.

After he had left he met a man in rehab who had also been at the unit. He mentioned one particularly gorgeous nurse. Ian said she was lovely, and the chap replied that Ian should have pursued it, "I had her in the linen cupboard." But with time, and increasing expertise, where there is a will . . . "Fumbling for buttons is difficult and you have to be more up front. Undoing bra fasteners at the back is impossible, you need front loaders if you buy her underwear. You adjust."

Since the illness Ian has been married three times and enjoyed each to the full. Though his intimate sexual life is private he agreed to allow some parts to be related, since the uniqueness of his condition allows important insights into function otherwise known only to him.

There is no reason to expect motor functions—erection and ejaculation—to be affected by the neuronopathy. Sensation, though, is different. Though he gets a pleasurable orgasmic rush with ejaculation, his peripheral sensation is diminished, though not abolished. This suggests that sensation over the penis may be a complex interaction between small and large sensory fiber function.[14] Sensation here is not a well worked out area, for understandable reasons of prurience which even scientists share, and because of the investigational difficulties. This is one reason why Ian's experiences are so valuable.

Imagine if your body felt no touch or movement and that you had to attend for any pain, fatigue, and occasional temperature sensations to guide it. Then imagine lying next to your loved one and feeling her or him next to you, from head to toe, your body now filled with sensations of warmth and proximity without any sensation of touch. Remember now that, for Ian, any sensation which is not pain becomes pleasure; imagine how precious these moments must be. Indeed they may be much more intense since then—and only then—through intimate temperature from another rather than intimate touch, can his body truly become alive sensorially. Intimacy, flesh to flesh, warmth to warmth, becomes enveloping and perhaps only then are sensation and feeling united, through and on the body; through warmth to pleasure. For Ian such sensations may be overwhelming. Ian, however, is careful to qualify this concentration on skin and sensory nerves alone. "It's not the sensation alone. Context is so much more important; this person has allowed me in. It is not just touch, but being allowed to touch; this is intimacy."

In the *Shorter Oxford English Dictionary* (1983), the definition of intimacy begins abstractly, almost cognitively: "Inmost, deep seated, hence essential; pertaining to the inmost thoughts or feelings." Only then does it become more social: "close in acquaintance or association, characterized by familiarity," before leading—possibly—to a more bodily definition; "pertaining to or dealing with close personal relations." In contrast, a modern on-line dictionary equates intimacy—completely—with a special friendship or attitude to another person or place; "the *intimacy* of old friends, the *intimacy* of their relationship, the band liked the *intimacy* of the nightclub." *Merriam Webster's* list of synonyms includes belonging, closeness, and familiarity. These encompass its common, present meaning, a special form of relation between a person and others or a place, and one which has a pleasant affective or emotional tone, and so implies mutuality and consent. It also has exclusivity; one can be intimate with a relatively small number of people or places—it may be diminished by being (over) extended.

To become intimate with someone else also, usually, tends to either be mediated through or focused on the body, and people with problems in and of their body have particular problems in this regard.[15] Ian has revealed something of the creative ways he has used to transcend these. But far more important in intimacy, neuronopathy or not, is the entering into, and maintenance of, relationships. Acts of personal intimacy, shared acts, shared sensations, are profound and personal ways of reducing the space between ourselves and others. And in those, Ian, so often separated from people by the needs of his neuronopathy, can become as one with another, like the rest of us.

NOTHING LOST

Following a seminar in the Bronx in around 1997, courtesy of Herb Schaumburg, Ian has done several presentations to a general audience. In April 2013 he talked at Oliver Sacks' 80th Birthday Festival at New York Live Arts and at the Institute of the Humanities, New York University, organized by Lawrence Weschler. By now Ian is a natural in front of an audience, and he had the New York audiences spellbound. During the first talk he explained:

> I was bloody minded and explored what I had left. I never understand the science; it does not really grab me. I am much happier just getting on with it. I was disembodied at the start, lost, and in the early stages needed everything done for me. The big thing was when I learned how to sit up by myself; that was the key, an absolute turning point in my rehabilitation and ultimately my life. Even now, I wake up and think, "Where am I in space?" Each day I need to gradually re-associate myself before moving. So, rather than being disembodied, I am completely, totally, embodied. If I was not I would not know where I am. I re-associate and reconnect constantly. Everything is through vision. I think about it, before I do it; I think it out and I think it back.[1]

One of Ian's supreme skills is to hide the sheer effort and attention he uses each day and each minute. His needs to be safe and to navigate through the world are reflected in the way in which he remembers going abroad, for instance. He remembers the precise details, years later, of stairs and steps, doors and distances. And when he has watched himself, in past research or in the *Horizon* documentary, his comments are not vague thoughts about what he was feeling, but precise analyses of his posture and why he made particular movements or gestures at a given time. Most of us move around with little awareness of what we are doing. In contrast Ian's immersion in the physicality of his body and the built environment is conscious and constantly vigilant:

> What made the haul so difficult was that I did not have the vocabulary to explain it. I had spent time talking to doctors but they did not know what it meant, to me.[2] The first doctor to ask how I live with it was Jonathan. He asked about the human side as well as the clinical; that was a revelation in those days. It is crucial to understand what it is like, and Jonathan was the first person to actually listen. I have met Oliver, and lots of scientists and other great men and women. The ones that stand out are those that listen.

I live at the edge; I chose to live at the best of my ability and accept that anything will knock me back. There is no reserve; a head cold and I go to bed, unable to think sufficiently to move.[3] OK, I have lost spontaneity. I have to plan, both my next move but also whether I have the energy to meet you next week. But I have had a long journey, met many interesting, amazing people along the way and been to some brilliant places. I don't think I have lost anything; I have gained a lot. No, I cannot walk up a mountain, but at the end of the day I have done other stuff. I would never have met the people at NASA, never met Peter Brook, or Oliver, gone to Germany, or Goteborg, which has enriched my life. My disability came with me for the ride and nudged me in different directions. I understand more about me. It is part of my life . . .

Thinking back, he has wondered why on earth he, being so private, cooperated not just in the science but in his biography and a TV program, which cost him anonymity. His second wife, Linda, raised the same question; for someone so private, why was he doing it?

I never came out with a good answer then, but looking back, when I met Jonathan, my first wife, Mavis, had died the year before and my journey was lonely. My early rehabilitation was known to me alone. The physiotherapists had their agenda and I worked to mine, private and alone, and the two did not really overlap. Later, I continued with college and then work, and for years did not discuss it with anyone. Mavis did not understand the nuances of my disability, but could see me for what I was. She encouraged me, understood me, and could read me; I had someone. When, suddenly, she was gone, I was alone, again.

I was intrigued that anyone thought I could contribute in the research area, and flattered. I went along with it, and when Jonathan started probing and asking unusual questions, I saw someone in a professional field who would understand and I could tell things to, a bit like a counselor, to gel with and discuss. From there it spun off into various directions and that, for me, has been the interesting part. That is why it started.

Pride and a Daily Marathon laid a few ghosts. It was cathartic since it was an opportunity to revisit things. But the process was not easy—literally. I say so much and yet so little comes out that is good enough for inclusion.

Ian has been working with scientists since the mid-1980s, when some neuroscientists he works with now were not yet born. One US professor said he was jealous of Ian, "His CV is better than mine; he has more papers."[4] Though initially cautious and passive in labs, he is now very experienced; his time as a "guinea pig" was short.[5] He takes research very seriously and works very hard letting researchers know how he has done a task. One never does an experiment *on* Ian but *with* him.

One of his initial frustrations was in comparisons with other deafferented subjects who might have done the same experiment. He soon learned to know when he entered a lab how good the science would be. He dislikes a department where the boss cannot be questioned. He prefers measured exploration during an experiment, with time for thought and further experiments, to an experiment with a single point to prove:

> Science, for me, is curiosity. I was always interested in movement; when that is taken away, suddenly, doing the research enabled me to understand a bit more about the loss and what it is, and more about the strategies to overcome it.

Though he accepts how powerful the Popperian science of falsifying hypothesis can be, his inclination—like that of many neuroscientists—is motivated by an informed curiosity.[6] He likes people thinking and questioning on their feet. He enjoys going to a lab and meeting the people who are almost invariably fascinated by his experience. But he feels he has to retain some distance, since he needs to perform scrupulously in experiments to make sure the science is right, and does not want familiarity, or loathing, to alter his motivation.

There is also another aspect to the science which can be difficult to tease apart. In some experiments subjects are passive, say when the brain's responses to a sensory stimulus are being recorded, and in others they are asked to make responses or movements, but these are stereotyped, constrained, and require little cognitive control, so that large numbers of control subjects will move the same way. But each time Ian moves he has to think about it and so it reflects his cognitive condition and a decision by him to move in a certain way. He may use one strategy one day and a different one the next. So it is always important to ask Ian exactly what he did and how he did it. This adds complexity to most experiments and led one eminent neuroscientist to suggest that experiments with Ian are the most demanding he has been involved in. This need for both more conventional third-person science and first-person involvement can be a problem, but is also one of the most stimulating aspects of working with Ian. Scientists, who are usually taught not to rely on a subject's introspection, to keep their distance, and to remain dispassionate for fear of compromising objectivity, have to be open to another way, especially since he has so much expertise.

This distance between first- and third-person perspectives was perhaps seen best in the experiments in Chicago with David McNeill. David was interested to read of Ian's concerns about the study isolating gesture in a lab rather than also looking at how he used it socially, during a meal or a beer:

> I now see, for the first time, how Ian was perceiving us on his visits here. He felt we were not paying sufficient attention to his own experiences and insights into his gestures. And not properly appreciating the effort, control, judgment, and discipline he has raised to get these gestures. And he is quite right. Partly, I think, because we had limited time and were focused on getting our tests carried out, but more, I realize now how much we were seeing the whole thing as a psych experiment, where the participant [Ian] and the experimenter have a constant distance. I suppose this rankled him the most.

Ian can accept being seen as a subject; he was more concerned by the impression he received of a preconceived idea about how he would "behave" or "respond," almost as though he was "a jigsaw piece to fit into their picture of things." David's evidence is carefully observed and built up, and to an extent was preconceived in relation to a hypothesis, as science should be. David continued:

> From your description, what I missed in Ian revolves around how he starts gestures; but there is nothing that he can do with intentions to have created the tight gesture–speech synchronies at points where gesture and speech are co-expressive; and this for me is the important point.
>
> I hope Ian does not think we are minimizing his achievements by saying that his gestures are normal. It is the timing of gesture and speech we are referring to, not the occurrence of the gesture itself, which I think Ian takes most pride in. The blind was crucial of course, since otherwise Ian would have had a way, visually, to keep speech and gesture together, and what we wanted to know, and could find out only from him, is whether they come together just by the fact of speaking itself. He may not realize how exciting it was for us to see his gestures and speech synchronized under the blind. It was as if we were touching the origin of language.
>
> I'm not surprised that gesture survived Ian's catastrophe. If he could speak it must have. Of course, he could and did control them. You're right too; those gestures from the start support the theory. Too bad we don't have films of him then. It would be most interesting to see if he also had gesture–speech synchrony—I bet he did.

Ian wants to explore a more natural, enriched, condition for gesture, when two or more people are chatting, with no awareness of being filmed, and when the normal turn-taking and ebb and flow of conversation unfolds. For him the most natural gestures, with least effort, are in casual social situations, and it is these he is most interested to analyze. His concern was that he might have exaggerated some gestures because he was being filmed by David and the BBC. One imagines that David, too, would like to be in a position to analyze these more natural gestures, but he needs to formalize his study material to be able make comparisons between participants. Without a set gestural narrative—the cartoon—David would have found it difficult to compare Ian with others and he would not have uncovered, in such beautiful detail and complexity, what gesture conveys and how it is constructed. And without the screen we could not have seen Ian's gestures without visual supervision. David continued:

> Another reason for experimenter neutrality is to avoid having the experimenter become a factor in the experiment. But of course this very stance was a factor for Ian. In spite of it all we saw very important things.[7]

Despite these concerns Ian is very pleased he was involved. "I enjoyed my time in Chicago and David is an amazingly dedicated and talented scientist." It is a measure of how much Ian was involved that he is still concerned to question and debate several years later.

He always does his best, regardless of whether he likes the lab and the people. Sometimes, though, it goes wrong. "There was, in one lab, an irritating tit. I could not have done what he asked me to do, so I did not waste my energy trying. If I cannot see a way to do it, then I cannot do it."[8]

For Ian, as for the rest of us, a movement has to be physically possible but also mentally possible. He has to structure it in his mind; it is about planning as well as doing. Remember those childhood games of patting the head and stroking the tummy in a circle? Neither on its own is problematic, but together they become difficult, as though the mental programs to do each movement cannot work together. Ian has to think how to do almost everything, every day, and conceptualizing movements can be very demanding and tiring.

On the other hand, very occasionally, he moves without being fully aware of what he is doing. When he first sat up in bed he moved his head up to see and then contracted his stomach muscles, but since he had never done that before, there was an element of doing before thinking; subsequently he went back to analyze exactly what he did. There are just a few occasions when even he is not sure how he did something. He once walked and remembers thinking not of walking but of where he was, something used by Peter Brook in L'Homme Qui. Ian also remembered work in Munich with Franz Mechsner and Wolfgang Prinz. "Go back to the experiment with the flags and the wheels. I did not have a clue how that was working, but I managed it."[9]

In this Ian sat at a table below which were two wheels he turned by rotating two hand-held cranks. He could see neither the cranks nor the wheels but could see two flags which rotated above the table in the same circular motion as the wheels below. Each time Ian circled a wheel underneath the table its flag went round once above it, and the two wheels and flags were the same. Ian could hold the cranks under the table and rotate his hands to make the flags circle without too much difficulty. Then Franz introduced a 3:4 gearing between one flag going round and the movement under the table, without telling Ian what had happened. For the flags to go round together now Ian had to circle one side three times to the other's four. It was no longer possible to relate hand position and flag position since they were changing the whole time. Probably for the first time since his illness, he had to let go of where he thought his hands were and control a transformed moving target, the flags. Ian had always controlled movement by thinking it through, and seeing where he was, or imaging it visually; now they were asking him to use an entirely different strategy. Though by no means perfect, Ian was able to do this for a short time, once Franz explained what was going on. He was able to move from a focus on his hand position to one on the transformed visual feedback to improve movement control. Ian was fascinated that he could do it and remembers the experiment years later, even though he is still not quite clear how he did it.

Ian is unaffected by becoming a "famous" subject. An irony is that the time when, arguably, he was most feted publically, with the Brook theater piece and the BBC *Horizon*, was also when he was living alone and not well off. It cannot have been easy rubbing shoulders with people at the National Theatre while wondering how he was going to make ends meet. But he would not have missed it for a moment; he thought *L'Homme Qui* was fabulous:

> Peter Brook was charming. If I had known how eminent he was I would have been more reverent. At the end of *L'Homme Qui* I said to him that there was no plot. He explained that theater did not always need one. It can educate and enthuse without. I was very grateful that he let us in on his rehearsal and his preparation methods, which are usually closed. I loved what he did. It was spooky, sitting in a public theater which was packed, watching myself portrayed when no one else knew . . .

That all seemed a long time ago, when Ian was more naïve and star struck. But then, as sometimes happens, the past resurfaced. Brook and his collaborator, Marie-Hélène Estienne have recently returned to neurology, 20 years after *L'Homme Qui. The Valley of Astonishment* focuses on synesthesia and derives in part from Alexander Luria's study of a man with a phenomenal memory. Their purpose, in part, is to see neurological conditions not as defect or deficit but as revealing something of the enhanced perceptual lives that those with synesthesia can lead. In an interview with Sarah Hemming, Brook said, "The people with this condition actually receive moments of their life more richly than we do. . . ." Within the play he has found space to explore a one-armed sleight-of-hand magician and to revisit Ian's case anew. Hemming introduced it thus:

> He talks about one man who lost his proprioception—the inner sense of body position that enables us to co-ordinate movement—and yet learned, painstakingly, to control his limbs again by using his eyes. Brook continued, "He came to see us when we were doing *The Man Who*. To everyone's amazement, the door of the theatre opened and he strode in, sat down and crossed his legs. We thought someone would have to carry him in from the taxi. But he says he cannot for one second let go of this acute attentiveness with the eyes. Even today. If, for a moment, the lights go out, he has learned how to let himself lean backwards against a wall because otherwise he would fall on the floor."
>
> "And the thing that is so moving is that for him the great joy of Christmas Day is that he is alone in his house and he sits on his chair and just lets himself go." Brook demonstrates, letting himself go limp. "Because every moment for him is a marathon. Every moment."
>
> Brook stops, clearly moved. And this surely is the nub of the show: it is not designed to make audiences gawp at case histories, but to alert them to the out-of-the-ordinary

capabilities of the mind. The piece encourages us to empathise with the characters but also to think about the perceptive tools we use to understand theatre. It's about awareness in several senses: about what it means to be human.[10]

When the company came to London's Young Vic to perform *The Valley*, Ian met them to assist Marcello Magni's portrayal of Ian. It was moving to see Peter and Ian meet again 20 years on, older but still questioning, with their mutual respect evident. *L'Homme Qui* had a dozen or more vignettes; that Peter had come back to Ian after this length of time, at this stage of his life, reinforced what an effect Ian had had on him and made this more than a portrayal. It was Peter honoring Ian before the world, not simply as a participant in neuroscience experiments, but as a person and as a spirit.

The new piece started with a doctor proclaiming a slightly updated account of Charles Bell's exposition of movement and position sense from his great *Hand* book of 1833, the first quotation in *Pride and a Daily Marathon*:

> There is inconsistency and something of the child's propensities still in mankind. A piece of mechanism, as a watch or dial will fix attention . . .; yet the organs through which he has a thousand sources of enjoyment, and which are in themselves more exquisite in design and more curious both in contrivance and mechanisms, do not enter his thoughts. We use the limb without being conscious, or at least, without any conception of the thousand parts which must conform to a single act . . . by an effort of the cultivated mind we must rouse ourselves to observe things and actions of which sense has been lost by long familiarity.[11]

Marcello then walked stiffly down from the side stall onto the stage and related his experience. At one point he leaned forward, cross-legged, cocked elbow resting on his knee, and head on hand, just like David Bennent had done, as he imitated Ian watching David portray him in a performance during the original production; an isolated gesture from one performance in Newcastle of *The Man Who* which has lived on for 20 years.

When *The Valley* was mentioned Ian was very interested to help and to meet Peter and the cast. He was humbled and flattered:

> Meeting Peter and Marie-Hélène again was very thought-provoking. Naturally we had all changed; Peter as pin-sharp and as insightful as I had remembered, Marie-Hélène as astute and perceptive as before but also more relaxed, and me now in a wheelchair.
>
> It was astonishing to see the new production. The thought that after 20 years they would have even considered using the original vignette again was humbling, but then to have developed it further and given it a new twist was astounding. After all Peter Brook and his company have undertaken and achieved in the intervening years, I am profoundly moved that they should have chosen my narrative from the original production. What an honor.

Having seen a run-through it was absolutely brilliant to meet the cast, and in particular Marcello who portrayed me. We joked about his dedication to detail as he, like me, was displaying a wide parting in his hair and a handsome moustache. I was deeply touched by his sensitive and sincere portrayal.

In fact it was a blast for Ian to sit afterwards in the theater café with Marcello and Kathryn Hunter, who played the synesthete and mnemonist, and swap stories and ideas. Ian was very happy with Marcello's portrayal, for the moustache and above all for its feeling and tone:

> I am often asked what is it like to see myself portrayed, and I have never found an easy answer, it is such a mixture of emotions-and weird. People paying to see the performance is bizarre. In the performance itself I have to accept that there are always elements I would like to tweak, it is the perfectionist or obsessive nature in me. But I can now accept it is an interpretation, an impression, and I am comfortable with that. Of course I would always like the opportunity to meet and engage with the actor before they portrayed me, but let us be realistic, that's not feasible. Marcello's portrayal is great; a very compassionate and considered interpretation.
>
> In TV programs such as *Horizon* or on radio, like most people, I have an aversion to seeing or hearing myself. Though I never have an opportunity to control the edit, so I can never be sure how the program will end up, at least it is me being me. I can only hope to portray my condition as best I can.
>
> These media pieces compare with *Pride* and, now, this *Losing Touch* escapade. Jonathan spends hours, days, years, researching, writing, editing, and then we sit to discuss, and I always read what is written. These written accounts may lack performance but they reach a depth rarely approached in other ways.

Ian had not heard of Peter Brook before he met him. In contrast, he was aware of Oliver Sacks, though he remained slightly skeptical:

> I didn't like the idea of the guy initially. Picking up people like me, making a story, and then leaving the subjects to get on with their lives. It did not help that when we met he was quiet and introverted.[12]

Ian's views changed over the years as he got to know Oliver:

> I sat by him once and said, "Oliver, you are eccentric," and Oliver replied that he was very aware that if he did not have a white coat and a name badge he'd not be let out of the asylum. Oliver had a great sense of humor.

Ian was not averse to manipulating him either. Once, preceding Oliver into their hotel in Houston, he noticed some cycads. Knowing of Oliver's love for them, Ian stopped and touched one, anticipating that Oliver would be unable to resist. Sure enough, Oliver asked Ian why he had stroked one, since he couldn't feel it. "I just wanted to engage with this shy, quiet, complex guy, and it was worth it."[13] That evening at dinner Ian sat close to Oliver, who remarked on how easily Ian engaged with people. "That is something I find difficult." Ian found it endearing that such a famous man should have been so honest, and self-deprecating:

> He may not have been as empirical [as some scientists], but he made it OK to explore conditions and to engage with those who have those conditions as people, not subjects, not objects, but as people. He has humanized what previously was pathologized and enriched us all along the way. We need more Olivers, not more researchers.

Considering the relation between intentional action and self, Samuel Beckett wrote, "You do what you are, you do a fraction of what you are, you suffer a dreary ooze of your being into doing."[14] This relation between being, thinking and doing was explored in a different perspective by Merleau-Ponty:

> Consciousness projects itself into the physical world and has a body . . . [it] is in the first place not a matter of "I think that" but of "I can." Consciousness is being-towards-the-thing through the intermediary of the body. . . . The body is the general medium for having a world. . . . my love, hatred and will are not certain as mere thoughts about loving, hating and willing: on the contrary the whole certainty of these thoughts is owed to that of the acts of love, hatred and will of which I am quite sure because I perform them. . . . I make my reality and find myself only in the act . . . It is not because I think I am, that I am. The whole certainty of love, hatred or will is that I perform them.[15]

Jonathan first quoted these words in relation to people who become tetraplegic; what sort of existence is lived when one cannot move below the neck? But this is also relevant to Ian, since all his movements are so deliberate and intentional, and why he tried so hard during his early rehabilitation to regain his body as a medium through which, in which, he could act and be, and so have a world. Since he has to think about movement so much more than other people, one can see his motor thoughts unfold; the closeness of thought to action is one reason why he found the experiments on gesture so interesting but also so revealing; they threatened to get close to who he was.

And yet Merleau-Ponty's conclusion is not entirely true; it is not only in the act that people exist. People who live with tetraplegia say that they can exist in other's actions, say those of their personal assistants who undertake tasks on their behalf. In a similar manner Ian talks of both his audits and his turkey work with equal passion and levels of interest and immersion. But whereas he does the hard work of an audit, observing and measuring, planning and composing reports, he can do little hands-on work with the turkeys. As Brenda says:

> Physically he cannot feed them; he can open the back doors to see into their houses, but he cannot handle them as grown birds. When they are young, he manages their incubation and can handle the new chicks until they are in the field. He does his access work and photography, but the turkeys he cannot do—though he is just as passionate. I don't get the passion, I just do the birds.

So, there is no difference in the way Ian talks of his audit work, which he is physically involved with, and the work with turkeys, geese, hens, and peacocks, which he is not. He is also developing a successful career writing "hands-on" articles in various animal husbandry magazines. None of his readers would realize he does not actually do what he writes about with so much knowledge, wisdom, judgment, and gentle humor.[16] Ian's reality, and hands-on journalism, is not solely in the act, it transcends his own movement to exist in others' actions and in his intentions, thoughts, plans, and enthusiasms.

We usually move with little thought to how we do it, our bodies just do what we want. We think about our goals rather than our movements; we do not think about where we put our legs, arms, and fingers when making tea, we just make it, having decided we want some. Indeed if we did think about our movements we would find it extraordinarily difficult to know everything we did.[17] Once Jonathan asked Ian, when sitting in a café, to describe his level of attention when reaching for a cup of tea:

> I am initially being aware of my body position to hang it all off. Sitting down my legs are in a tripod, sitting on a chair, and I have a mental image of this. Having my arm resting on the table is a good triangle position, and I know I can then reach the cup. Once the framework is safe and I can monitor hand out and in, then I can begin. I see it all except what the fingers are doing behind the cup, but I have learned to do this [by grasping without using the handle]. I don't know how heavy the cup is, so pick it up and monitor it visually. I need to see my arm up to my face, but then I can feel the cup with my face. I may not need to see the cup return until it reaches the table. This is all very controlled and involved.

Firstly Ian has to want the tea sufficiently to make the effort of movement worthwhile. Then, before making any movement, he rehearses it in his mind, his "pre-visualization." The effort involved in these movements is very tiring, and tiredness, in turn, affects his ability to think sharply enough about movement:

> I cannot concentrate on all aspects of walking. In a given movement, say from here to the door, a distance of 20 feet, I think two steps ahead roughly. If it is busy I will sit and wait. Walking is never the same each time. I apply the strategy which is easiest at the time. These are not always major changes but, like a snooker player,

some days I have flair and some days not. It is a very lonely path. There is no familiarity with the others I have met with the same condition; we are so different in this regard.

Inner achievements are all; goal setting, pre-visualization. I cannot be too intellectual about it though, because all my intellectual effort is in doing, not in reflecting on it. I can't spend too long thinking about it, because if I thought what I have to do all my life I would be too scared.

Elements of movement are easier because I have the confidence or arrogance in my abilities. When a bird learns to fly it leaves the nest and goes sit on a branch, and its expectation is that the branch won't break; it trusts the branch. To become mobile and live independently I have learned to manage a range of movements, and I trust my ability to choreograph them in a way that I want. That's the payoff for all the hours, weeks, and months of training, an implicit self-belief; that my branch won't break.

Such "confidence" is difficult to investigate, dissect, or even describe. Ian thinks each movement into action and assumes it will unfold, with visual supervision. His link between the imagination and formulation of movement and action always involves risk and uncertainty. While he has described the mental effort of moving as a daily marathon, it is one performed on a high wire. He lives with levels of vulnerability that are difficult to comprehend.

The 2014 work of the eminent UK modern choreographer Siobhan Davies, *Table of Contents*, is a live performance created by her with five other dancers. They perform several pieces as they meditate on the relation between remembering and performing movements, between thought, memory, and action. The pieces take place in a space shared between performers and audience, with people able to come in and out as they like over the several hours it takes to unfold.

There are two pieces which are directly traceable to Ian's influence. In one, *To Hand*, Matthias Sperling moves round the floor spread-eagled and supported on upturned clear plastic pots. Every movement involves risk, as he balances, and thinks out the next movement and how he can manipulate his body in new ways. For some this is bewildering; a man lying down, balancing and moving on small pots for several hours; his attention focused not on a goal—say reaching the other end of the room—but more on the constituent parts of each movement. However as a graphic illustration of something of what Ian and many people with physical conditions go through each day it is compelling.

The second piece is simple yet startling. One of the troupe lies on the ground and invites a member of the audience to instruct them—through words—to stand. The performer moves exactly as told to; no more, no less. As Charles Bell wrote in 1833:

When a blind man, or a man with his eyes shut, stands upright ... by what means is it that he maintains an erect position? It is obvious that he has a sense by which he knows the inclination of his body and that he has a ready aptitude to adjust it. . . . In truth we stand by so fine an exercise of this power, and the muscles are, from habit, directed with so much precision and with an effort so slight, that *we do not know how we stand* [italics added].[11]

We can stand from lying easily, without thought. But it is extraordinarily difficult to analyze exactly what we do and to put that in words to instruct someone else to do it. Siobhan related what happens in the performance:

After the first nervous requests the member of the audience becomes intrigued by the difficulty of the task and notices that language doesn't help as much as they thought. There is a measure of frustration, curiosity, and pleasure, and it normally takes at least 15 minutes to complete the task. People learn to attend to the simplest of actions, common to us all. No one can describe the enormous ensemble of actions, and counter actions, needed to do this maneuver.

We were interested in how Ian would approach the task. One slight snag was that it was not a movement he is familiar with since he does not get down on floors. Initially Ian sat in his chair to instruct Matthias but soon decided he would have to lie down on the floor too, to refresh himself about the act in order to describe it. His method was to lift his head up and then contract his stomach muscles to rise to a seated position, then to cross his legs in front of him. Then, he asked Matthias to turn his torso to the left, and place his hands on one side on the ground. They took the weight as he asked Matthias to move his legs, one at a time, from their crossed position to underneath his body, in a compact squat. With feet, legs, and body turned to the side, in line with his hands on the floor, Ian asked Matthias to straighten his legs, lift his hands and arms from the floor, and stand. Though at times Matthias was skeptical, it worked.

Matthias soon realized the differences between Ian and naïve subjects:

Immediately and wonderfully apparent for me was the marked difference of working with someone who already *has* their own highly developed, readily accessible personal "manuals" for consciously accomplishing deconstructed everyday movements, rather than someone who is searching them out and attempting to break down a given movement for the first time. The second thing was simply how good his "manuals" were; how efficient, robust, effective, well-planned, streamlined, architecturally sound . . .

"Architecturally sound;" in a way Ian is an architect of his movements, planning and watching them unfold rather than being immersed in them like the rest of us:

The route we took was quite different from others; direct and confident. Ian instructed me to execute movements that most people would consider too dangerous or unlikely to be worth attempting, when in fact they are highly efficient solutions to the problem.

An example was the move into a squat (weight on two feet) from kneeling on one knee, stabilized by two hands also on the ground. It required quite a large adjustment of one part of the body, that could have led to toppling over unless well-stabilized, but that was exactly what was needed. Similarly, Ian's foreknowledge of where a given path would lead meant that many problems encountered along the way by most people, were avoided by forward planning.

Matthias was also struck by what he called the "design level" of Ian's instructions, neither the largest nor the smallest possible scales of deconstruction of movement, but somewhere close to the mid-point between these. This appeared to be the most effective use of energy, with an integration of complex information into useful composites and with reasonable durations of movement in each part. Matthias also noticed that Ian was more aware than others of the synergies required between parts of the body:

> Rather than working with a passive body, with no effort anywhere but in the part being instructed, Ian seemed to assume a body in which effort or activity remains more widely dispersed, even while attention to precision is more specifically targeted.

Here Ian is aware of what happens to the physics of the body in movement. Finally, Matthias was struck by Ian's mention of "belief" in a movement's possibility as an absolutely necessary prerequisite for performing that movement: "'Acts of belief,' in a very wide and embodied sense, are of ever greater interest to me as a fundamental way of understanding artistic activity."

Siobhan was impressed by the similarities between her world of performance and choreography and Ian's solitary world:

> He felt so much like any one of us in how he thinks about the concept, strategies, opportunities that movement gives us. We deal with movement as an investigation and so does Ian, but he has had to do this at an extraordinary life-supporting level. Matthias and I have chosen to do this but can leave the damn investigation when we want. His attention to *Manual* was imbued with all the empathy and consideration of one movement analyst and human being working with another. I know there is such an enormous difference in how our interest in movement came to pass but for a while, in the studio, we were there in the mix together and that felt right. I can't help but be moved by how much Ian has invested in movement as a way for him to live as he should, by his massive attention to BE in the world with us as equals while knowing all the time how much he has to DO in order to achieve that.

Ian does not willingly expose himself to dangerous environments in or outside labs. Occasionally, though, he is reminded of his continuing vulnerability. Illness can test his mental resources; the other constant is the need for light. He usually has back-up sources of lights around him, but can be found short, even at home. Recently he mentioned he had had a bad night; a bulb had gone and his back was a bit sore. On asking for more detail it came out . . .

> About quarter to ten I came into the lounge and switched the light on. The bulb went and it tripped all the electricity off. Brenda was working in Jersey so I was by myself. Immediately I thought, "I need to be safe." I was safe in my chair as long as I was in the same position, but I could not do that for 6–7 hours till it was light again.

He got to his office by turning his wheelchair, going through two narrow doorways and a short hall; on the way he bashed a table and knocked a pot plant off. The lap top was still on and from the glow he could see where he was. Then the screen saver came on, too dark for ambient light, so he had to tap around the desk surface to get it back on. He unplugged the laptop and, with it on his lap, used its glow to navigate back into the kitchen where there was a box of matches and a candle, kept for such emergencies. Except they had been moved. Eventually he found a candle, lit it, and then, by its light, lit a fire in the lounge; more light. But he needed to find the box of candles, since the fire and candle would burn out within the hour:

> I needed to phone someone to re-set the trip switch. The fuse box was beyond the kitchen, down a step and high on the wall. I could not reach it. I used to be able to do it with a broom handle but that is beyond me now.

One disaster came after another. He had arranged to change his mobile phone 2 days before, and was still waiting for a replacement. All his phone numbers were on the main computer, without power, so he was without phone numbers or internet.

> So, I was stuck with a candle which was burning down, a laptop running out of power, a fire which was burning out, and my home phone which was without power. Otherwise it was a fun evening.

He knew that the safest place was in his car where there was light, but was unsure how to get to it. His torch was in the footwell of the Gator [his electric buggy] he used to get round the fields, parked just outside the door. If he put the candle on the window sill and if he timed it when there was no cloud, he could reach to the Gator, by the light of the moon, switch it on, and get to the car. Then he remembered the fuse had gone on the Gator lights:

> I put the candle on the door step and got out of my parked wheelchair, and then I got stuck. There is a small step outside the house, of 3 inches or so, which I normally step

over without a problem. This time I froze half way during the transfer; the worst thing for me. Usually I get started and the momentum carries me through a movement to keep it going. The hardest thing is to stop half way and then reinitiate the movement. I got exceedingly tense and had strong pain in the lower back. Somehow I fell into the Gator, managed to turn round and get into the seat. I had a torch, so I had light. But the batteries were not freshly charged and I knew I had to get to the car.

In the house Ian had used the car keys to open the car remotely, to see how long it stayed open with the lights on. He realized that he would probably not have time to get to the car from the Gator. He had to try it, however, and lurched to the car and pulled the door handle. He hoped the door would open and the lights go on, but, sure enough, it had self-locked. He had the torch and keys in the same hand, since he needed the other hand to open the car. So next he tried to unravel that hand to find the button to press the fob to open to car. In the end, he put the torch on the floor with the keys in front of it and pressing the fob down onto the ground, using his other hand to steady himself against the car. Then he opened the car door and sat in with a huge sigh of relief. Once the key was in the ignition, he had light. He had thought he would use the car phone to get Fishy Pete's number from directory enquiries, except he turned out to be ex-directory:

> By now I thought I just needed some razor blades to finish it. I tried his son, the only number I had, but no answer. So I left the house open, the candles burning, and the log fire going and set off for Axminster, 5 miles away, to Fishy Pete's.

Pete lived on a one-way system, in a terraced house with no pavement, with his door and window on the road. The trouble was that it was on the wrong side of the road. He had no stick to lean across and hit the door or window, and he couldn't get out the car because, by now, his back was so sore. He drove round the one way system a couple of times hoping to meet someone to ask them to knock on his door:

> That would have been an interesting conversation past 11 o'clock at night, but I saw no one. So I drove, slowly, the wrong way round the one way system so my car was pointing the other way, wound down my window and tapped on his window and he came to the door. We were back at my house within 15 minutes. He hit the trip switch and all the lights came back on.

What Ian did not say was that he had tapped on the window by throwing bananas at it, the only things to hand in the car. Fishy Pete has never let him forget that. Once back in the house and safe he was so wound up that he could not sleep. The incubators, with 2000 turkey eggs, had been off for 2 hours or more ruining many of the eggs.

Next day an electrician re-sited the trip switch and installed another circuit. Normally Ian would have torches all round the place but he had got a bit complacent:

Even I take it for granted that I have movement and mobility, but in darkness it was all gone and I am just as helpless now as I was all those years ago. I have all those strategies, but the key to making them all work—other than a brain—is vision. If I cannot see, then I cannot do anything. It made me realize how vulnerable I am, even after all these years. It was not the best evening.

Ian and Jonathan met Jacqueline McCoy and her husband in New York in 2013. Thirty years previously, when she was 33, she developed a neuropathy after diarrhea with severe sensory loss of both touch and proprioception. Unlike Ian, she could always feel sharp, and indeed is hyper-sensitive; smooth is cool, roughness unpleasant. Her wedding ring hurt her finger and she had her legs shaved because the stubble hurt. Right from the beginning she visualized everything in order to move. She was in hospital for a month and then went to a nursing home for rehab. Six weeks later she cooked for her family and soon after that she stood.

She still walks, despite falls, has tried golf with her husband, been on a Mediterranean cruise with a girlfriend, and while in New York walked the mile or so to Ground Zero. But recently she had noticed her energy levels reducing. She used to do a full day's work, be a hockey mom, and then do the laundry. Now she gets tired, her walking is less accurate, and she has broken toes hitting things. Her main reason for coming to New York from Florida was to ask Ian if he had ideas about how she could adapt as she got older.

For once Ian was silent. He had often said that since he lived at his peak he would have to slow down as he aged, just as athletes have to live with reduced performance. But quite how he did not know. The wheelchair was the big thing:

As I have aged I am more chilled out. Ever since I developed strategies to walk I have been aware that it may not go on forever, that I may not put all the building blocks together to move. Now my back is painful much of the time, because of how I have walked. Aside from that, I can get round in a wheelchair. That is a fact of life. I was never happy about the chair, but I can do my work more effectively from it. It was hard, but I have done it now. You have to compromise. One of the big things for me was financial. I go round stores and banks auditing them. I could no longer do that walking. I do it from a wheelchair, or I don't eat. Being in a chair does not affect how clients see me, quite the reverse. I do a better job and see more. The wheelchair was a big change in my life, I really do better and see more.

If I was presented with the same situation now, I probably would not work as hard to walk. I would want to transfer independently, maybe manage steps, and be a bit mobile, but the world has moved on, it's more accessible. I did what I felt was right for me at the time, and I don't regret not going into a chair earlier, and I certainly don't regret a single moment of the effort and time I spent walking. But I do regret being so hard on people, and especially my mum, who tried to encourage me into a chair years ago.

The other side is the cognitive effort of putting all these tricks and strategies together to move . . . how long will I be able to do that? I have lost energy and capacity. I still have to think about not falling out of the chair and leaning forward . . . I still think about dexterous movements . . . will I still string them together? More and more I find a distraction, say a cold, makes it harder to plan and construct movements and strategies. It is becoming more taxing; another fact of life. The strategies I have applied over the years have not become any easier, even though I use them every day. I use the analogy that my movements are made up of smaller ones which I join together to make an action. The alphabet, words, sentences have never been second nature. It has never got easier, never will. Making sentences from letter and words has got harder and I put that down to age.

Brenda also mentioned how being in a wheelchair allows him to see more. In shops, for example, she does not have to look out for him; quite the reverse, she can lose him as he goes off on his own:

Ian going into a chair took the stress away. I was always looking round to see what might happen. Being purely selfish, it takes a lot of work out of going places. Now that worry has gone.

They live beside a forest and, now he has a motorized chair Brenda cannot keep up. He goes out for 3 or 4 hours off track, into a whole new world for him:

When I was totally absorbed in being mobile and just standing, I missed so much. Now for work, and for my social life and recreation, the wheelchairs are a real blessing. They free up mental energy and I can have more social life and take on more work.

But the chairs were not the whole answer:

What happens when I get older? Will I still make the connections? I do have worries; I am not sure how I will manage. I think I will still be able to do all the feeding and dressing stuff, but it will take longer.

However Ian manages the next part of his life he will do it with the same invention, creativity, humor, and stubbornness with which he has lived for the last 40 years or so. And he will do it with the admiration and affection of a huge number of local friends and of grateful scientists around the world.[18] His single-handed and single-minded contribution to the understanding of proprioception and touch has been extraordinary, and is recognized by many scientists. Herb Schaumburg described his feelings thus:

Those not in the field do not appreciate what he has achieved through hard work, dedication, and what I characterize as a triumph of the will. I never realized what it was till I encountered Ian. To never ever stop thinking about what you are doing and to be so motivated as to do that, generally people just give up.[19]

Herb was speaking literally; without conscious attention to movement—his will—Ian cannot move, and would not have done for the last 40 years or so. But also "will" in the more usual meaning, to impose oneself on what one does. His discipline in thought and action has enabled him to do all that he has. He has married three times, picked himself up from bereavement, and from being unemployed twice, learned two new areas of work and interest, and excelled in both. During this he has also spent many days and weeks assisting scientists selflessly, so that they might understand proprioception and movement more. And all the time he has been a life-enhancing presence, enriching those around him with the simple joy of living and a humor not easily explored in print.

As mentioned at the beginning of this chapter, in 2013 Ian was invited to talk at Oliver Sacks' 80th Birthday Festival in New York. Modest as ever, Ian was thrilled:

> I do the research hoping I might be contributing to an understanding of an aspect of movement and management of the body, which I hope is not a bad achievement. I viewed my invitation to his 80th Festival as an acknowledgement of this and though my input was actually quite small, I felt that to be asked at all was humbling and amazing. I was enormously grateful.

After the talk Ian found this online, from "Matt," a man at the workshop:

> On April 17th of 2013, I had the great pleasure of going to a talk about Ian's incredible story, with Ian as one of the speakers. What really struck me was just how natural Ian looked speaking with his hands, something I do unconsciously. For Ian, every motion, no matter how small must be thought, planned, and executed with conscious precision. Even a wayward gesture could throw him off balance and onto the floor.
>
> When asked why he would take such a risk, Ian replied simply, "Because appearing normal is important to me." This speaks to just how powerful our collective culture can be. This man must constantly live on the edge of his abilities just to stay upright, but he inches ever closer to that edge to create the appearance he values.
>
> After I left the talk I waited for my friend in the lobby, and Ian came by. I thanked him graciously for a wonderful talk, and Ian thanked me for the kind words. As he spoke Ian ever so gently reached out to touch my arm affirmingly. I know that Ian could not feel when he touched me; he could not even feel himself. Despite that, he must have felt it was important to show me he cared with this gesture. I was (and still am) emotionally quite taken by this experience.
>
> If Ian were rude, mean, and depressed I don't think many people would blame him. Every single day for him is a tremendous challenge. Yet Ian seems to embrace this challenge with kindness, courage, and a sense of humor. We could all probably stand to learn a thing or two from Ian.[20]

We could, and have.

AFTERWORD: PERSONAL PERSPECTIVES

One winter's day in 2014, rain everywhere, Jonathan drove to Dorchester station to pick up Arko Ghosh, who had flown in from Zurich, and Jack, a PhD student from University College London, and took them the 20 miles to Ian's house. Brenda had baked, so the first thing was tea, cake, and chat. Then they did the experiment, on the Kohnstamm phenomenon, in Ian's sitting room and at his kitchen table.[1]

Between experiments Ian was jocular and relaxed, during them completely focused. Once finished and packed up Jonathan drove Arko and Jack back to the station. As they were motoring back Jack asked if Ian was always that cheerful, and so full of life and interest. The answer was yes.

In writing about the ways in which the science behind various papers was done and revealing something of Ian's life over the last 25 or more years, Jonathan has tried not to invade Ian's privacy too much, nor to over-personalize the account. Just as Ian has talked of walking a knife-edge between friendship and objectivity when going to a lab, so Jonathan has navigated between affection and experiments. But it is impossible not to form a friendship with Ian.

In *Pride and a Daily Marathon* Jonathan quoted Oliver Sacks' re-formulation of Nietzsche, from the epilogue to *Awakenings*:

> Only great pain compels us to descend to our ultimate depths . . . I doubt such pain makes us 'better', but I know it makes us more profound. One returns with merrier senses, with a second innocence in joy more childlike and yet a hundred times subtler than . . . before.
>
> There are some hells known only to neurological patients. Those who return are forever marked by the experience. The effect to make them not only deep but child-like, innocent and gay . . . they survived . . . as figures made great by their endurance, for being . . . undaunted and finally laughing . . . maintaining an inexplicable affirm-ation of life.[2]

This still has resonance, but is not entirely apposite. Ian "returned" 43 years ago; he has been impaired for twice as long as he lived without the neuronopathy. As he has said many times, his present condition is his "normal." And "return" suggests a recovery or lessening of the loss, whereas he has to live with it now, each day, as he did all those years ago. He has also descended to his own hells several times since the illness stripped him of ease in movement and touch—when his first wife Mavis died, and when he was divorced and unemployed. These latter events were as threatening, or nearly as much, as the original diarrheal illness. Each time Ian has hauled himself back, and each time recovered his appetite for life.

One of the most precious gifts in life is to celebrate and relish the everyday. Ian loves to sit in a café and just watch how people move around in their lives; he wants to know all the gossip, with humor and generosity of spirit. Chat to Ian and he cheers you up. Children, sheep, turkeys, work, forthcoming trips, the muck heap opposite, he can chat about them all. Whether at High Table in an Oxford college, talking with scientists, or chatting in a café with friends, Ian is always the same; fascinated, generous, and full of humor. In *Pride and a Daily Marathon* Jonathan also quoted Wittgenstein (and Richard Feynman): "Humour is not a mood, but a way of looking at the world."[3] Ian looks at the world with humor, with openness and generosity to those around, and with a relish for the off-beat and the quirky eccentricities and personalities of those who pass through his life.

This is all the more remarkable given his constant and continuing need to attend to movement and posture and to predict any danger around him. Robert Murphy, who became tetraplegic late in life, wrote of how, "there is a balance between the falling back into ourselves and a need to reach out ... Amongst the disabled the inward pull becomes compelling, often irresistible ..."[4] Ian reaches out to others, engaging despite his need to monitor movement and coordination each and every second.

In this book we have followed Ian from callow lab rat to experienced and refined subject, and critic of science and scientists, (though it must be said that Jonathan has tempered some of his more acidic reflections on some neuroscientists). In the pursuit of balance, Jonathan also asked some of the scientists and others for their reflections on Ian as a subject coming to their labs.

The first point that came up again and again was Ian's contribution to the science itself. The two scientists who have worked with Ian most on the CT afferent work covered in Chapter 10 responded independently, but curiously similarly. Francis McGlone from Liverpool John Moores University said:

> I was working in industry when I first heard of Ian, leading a research group interested in the mechanisms underlying pleasant touch of the skin. When Ian found out where I was working at the time—a personal products company involved in among other things soaps—I was immediately saddled with the epithet "Suds!" This set the tone between us as it forewarned me that Ian has an ability to "cut to the quick" with his knife-sharp wit, and as I got to know him better I became very aware that my scientific interest would get nowhere until it had passed muster by him.

He was relentless and remorseless in his attempts to pull any ideas apart, necessary, I came to understand, since he had been treated in the past just like a "guinea pig" by researchers who did not see Ian at all, just a "condition" to be exploited by self-interested clinicians and scientists. Once the grilling was over—and this always resulted in a far improved experimental protocol—Ian was the perfect "lab-rat." His insightful and analytical mind added subjective information about his experience of affective (pleasant) touch.

Håkan Olausson, now in Linköping, also made the point that Ian gives as good as he gets, with humor as well as a keen eye for science:

Human volunteers taking part in research have commonly been referred to as "subjects." However, lately there has been a shift in the scientific literature where "participant" is used to stress the critical contribution from these volunteers, without whom the studies would have been impossible. "Participant" implies a more willing contribution than the more passive connotations of "subject." However, in most cases I think human volunteers are truly "subjects" rather than full participants, partly because they usually have no say in the design and conclusions of an experiment. In human research ethics the word "guinea pig" is probably unheard of.

Ian Waterman is neither a "guinea pig," nor a "subject." He is one of the few who fulfills all philosophical criteria for being called a "participant." I have been working with Ian for a decade, and I have learned to double the time I would normally schedule for experimentation since Ian will have a plethora of suggestions for improvement of the procedure and lengthy discussions about alternative explanations of the results. I am grateful, since in the end he always turns out to be right.

During a meeting in Britain, I spilt a full mug of coffee on the new carpet in Dr Cole's prestigious chief-of-physician's office, my eyes having been too intently fixed to a computer screen. I was embarrassed, Dr Cole desperately tried not to be upset, while Ian laconically commented that only a "subject" who relies on proprioception would make the mistake of putting a full mug of coffee on a surface that is tilted. Now, who's the "guinea pig"?

David McNeill's response stressed, once more, the fundamental importance he attaches to Ian's experience of gesture:

Jonathan Cole has described my epiphany in Paris, when I suddenly saw that speaking and gesturing were one "thing." Ian is the source of a second epiphany. I don't suppose he knows this.

When I met him at our first session in Chicago, I had read Jonathan's *Pride and a Daily Marathon* and knew something of how Ian had taught himself to control his movements in a completely new way—planning, thinking, intuitively calculating force, speed and trajectory; monitoring his body through the corner of his eye. Nothing, I thought, could be more different from the unconscious "just happens" movements I experience.

But when we met his gestures seemed to be of two kinds. Some indeed looked carefully planned, just as I had imagined. Ian paused before making them, watched his hand (usually the left), and wound up with his hand carefully back at rest. In a word, these gestures were "presented," "staged."

But others were not like that at all. These others were small, rapid, modulated on the fly, not looked at and perfectly synchronous with his speech—in a word, "unconscious," just like my own. Here was something interesting! The gestures of this second kind were untouched by Ian's aproprioception. They formed an unbreakable unity with his speech and, as such, needed neither proprioception nor careful staging. Ian would talk and they were just there. And here was my epiphany. These gesture–speech units were put there by language itself and how it evolved. That, for me, was a great insight Ian had brought that day in Chicago: in him we glimpse something of what was created when language began.

Chris Miall is a professor in Birmingham who works on motor control, the area in which most research has been done with Ian over the years, starting in Oxford:

I first met Ian in about 1993, having known Jonathan since 1982. Jonathan was then looking for scientists who were interested in testing Ian, arguing, rightly, that by understanding how Ian was able to control his movements without sensory inputs we would also understand the normal motor system better.

Ian arrived for experiments, and I got my first insights into the challenge—and the enormous fun—in testing him. We were measuring Ian's wrist movements, to see the effect of short delays between movements on his accuracy, and using a modified joystick that could record wrist flexion and extension. We also had Perspex, bits of paper, a good deal of sticky tape, and a lot of coffee to keep us going. We improvised as we went along, trying to ensure that Ian was comfortable with the tasks we asked him to do, and more importantly, trying to match his standards, as he told us exactly where our experiments were failing—for example where he could see some part of his hand or arm that we thought we had blocked from view. That first visit has set a pattern of working—we set up what we think may work, and we spend the day or days of his visits testing, modifying, and often rewriting our computer programs late into the evening.

But it is also a time when Ian reflects on what he's been doing, and can sometimes tell you how he has changed his strategies in order to do better. This is can be frustrating, as one cannot be sure the Ian tested one day is the same Ian the next day—if he finds a better way to do the task, he takes it. And it also a time in which I am continually confounded by the thought that as he sits there, comfortably chatting with us, he is without sensation and moving a body that he cannot feel—something that I suspect very few of us can appreciate.

So, after about 20 years, do I understand the human motor system better? Yes, probably. Do I understand Ian's performance—yes, a bit, but not nearly well enough.[5]

The difficulty in doing good science with Ian was also picked up by Patrick Haggard, a cognitive neuroscientist from UCL, who worked with Chris in those early days:

I've always had the impression that Ian tells us what to do. He knows something that we really don't. The classic model of a laboratory experiment involves the experimenter instructing the participant what to do, but we should really be more humble.

Ian cheerfully informed us that he could and did use his preserved temperature sensation to work out how he was moving, even though he had no position or movement sense. So I learned that the first experiment with Ian doesn't really work. The first experiment is about him telling you how to do a good experiment with him. He tells you what he does. You spend a long time thinking about it, and then, if you're lucky, you come up with a better experiment which really challenges him.

On one of Ian and Jonathan's first visits to London they were met by Geoff Barrett, whose lab they were visiting. Ian and Jonathan got out the car and Geoff asked, "Where's Ian"? He could not fit the man standing before him to the person with the neuronopathy. Brian Day from Queen Square, made the same point when he first met Ian, years later:

> We had arranged that Jonathan would bring Ian to my lab to do some experiments on his vestibular system. As I looked down Queen Square I saw two figures approaching, one of whom was Jonathan. I assumed the other was Ian but as I watched him walk towards me I wondered whether that could be true. He seemed to be walking too easily and well, albeit with a slightly stiff-knee gait. Just before he reached me, I said hello and held out my hand to shake his in greeting. He said nothing, walked straight past me, reached the door, held onto the handle, swiveled round and then held out his hand. Then it struck me—he was so totally engaged with the act of walking he was unable to perform that balancing act and shake my hand at the same time. Welcome to the world of Ian.

It is not only neuroscientists who remember Ian well. Peter Brook remembers:

> In preparing *The Man Who*, our work with the actors was above all improvising the behavior of different neurological conditions to understand them not in words but through direct physical experience. The case of Ian fascinated everyone and a long process began of trying to make real the first actions of moving and guiding the limbs with the eyes. We heard that Ian could visit us in rehearsal in Paris and one day the cast was sitting in the Bouffes du Nord, waiting expectantly. A member of the staff was outside to tell us when a taxi arrived and we were all mobilized and ready to run to help.
> Then suddenly, the doors flung open and a tall figure strode confidently into the acting area, sat down, and crossed his legs. It was Ian. He at once joined the group in exercises led by our Japanese actor Yoshi Oida. For all who worked entirely with feeling and sensation of the body, it was hard to believe that Ian was totally in command, with no sensation at all. From then on, Ian became for us a warm, human friend, to be watched and followed with admiration.

Emma Crichton-Miller, the producer of the BBC *Horizon* documentary "The Man Who Lost His Body," found working with Ian

> Both a revelation and a privilege. We could not have understood nor conveyed so much to the audience without Ian's heroic contribution.

She continued by pin-pointing something Ian is well aware of but rarely shares:

> He has made himself the master of a condition that threatens, at every moment, to master him. Through a tremendous intellectual effort he has become the most articulate observer of his own plight.
>
> From the first occasion when we met Ian, we recognized both his vulnerability and his astonishing achievement. Through his insights viewers were given intellectual possession of a faculty of which they may have been barely aware and which they take completely for granted. None of us will ever forget Ian. His dignity was married to great modesty. While the stress to him was huge, he managed almost all the time to make it appear gracefully effortless.

Ian's influence extends beyond neuroscience research and theatrical portrayal. He has studied movement with an intensity and a precision that few, if any, have done, whether neuroscientist, dancer, or even musician. Some years ago Jonathan was invited to talk at a Gulbenkian Foundation workshop in London. Also talking was a woman who spoke of dance and movement, from an expressive artistic perspective, so beautifully and elegantly that Jonathan overcame his usual shyness and introduced himself to her. Since then they have become friends. Siobhan (Sue) Davies is a dancer, choreographer, and movement expert of rare originality. She is quite clear how important Ian has been to her work and thoughts:

> Soon after I began to dance I heard a radio program which nominated alternative wonders of the world. One man did not choose a construction; instead he offered a movement—our human ability to balance on the small surfaces of our feet while walking. Before I heard this I had taken this extraordinarily complex organization for granted. When Jonathan told me of Ian I was astounded.
>
> Much of a dancer's work elaborates on the traditional capacity for us to receive information through a series of sensual feedbacks, the base lines for endless explorations. So I find Ian's situation powerfully moving. Not only because finding his body moment to moment must be exhausting but also because our bodies are part of our expression.
>
> He has to have a concept of what he is about to do, ahead of every move; where his energy, weight, balance, trajectory, and resolve are and how his movements might be read by someone else. He is like many dance artists for whom movement serves a practical and expressive purpose. The way in which he has had to re-gain his skills has helped me to appreciate more the exquisite orchestration of our everyday actions; his attention to everyday movements has impacted on how I have been re-thinking my relationship to dance making.

Mark Mitton is a magician with an intense interest in neuroscience. For Mark, magic involves manipulating the audience's visual attention, so they do not see his "magic," coupled with exquisite motor control. His skills are breath-taking and unbelievable. His appreciation of Ian's achievement in movement is that of a fellow magician and expert in action. His perspective also allowed a new way of looking at Ian's gesture:

> In my twenties, I spent 5 years as an apprentice to Slydini, a master of physical misdirection admired by magicians all over the world. One of Slydini's breakthrough discoveries was the creation of gestures that did not appear to be intentional. With this rare technique, one can pick something up and set it down, and the actions can be seen, yet not noticed.
>
> When Ian and I met, our discussion centered on a simple question: why do people notice or not notice certain gestures? We had both spent years thinking about human actions, what they tell people about our intentions, and how to use this information effectively. As a magician, I only need to create apparently unintentional actions to make magic tricks stronger. Ian works very hard on creating natural-looking gestures to interact with people in his everyday life. This was fascinating.
>
> Two days later, at a party for participants at the conference, I performed magic tricks with Ian and made it look as if he was the magician. I started secretly passing objects to him, and it was then that I first sensed the unique rhythm of his actions and that he has a completely different way of handling space and time. When you pass someone an object, they usually meet you halfway. Both parties take their proprioception for granted as their hands maneuver towards each other. But Ian's hand would not even start to move until mine had stopped, so that he had a specific target in space at a specific time. During the tricks, as I passed him objects under the potential scrutiny of the audience, I could feel how he goes through life carefully planning each gesture as he makes it. This is something he lives with but is impossible to see usually because he is so strong at mimicking how the rest of us move, and it was an extraordinary experience.
>
> Ian distinguishes three types of gestures: closed, open, and descriptive. He explained that most of his gestures would start as a movement towards a fixed point. Because their path is contained, he calls these *closed gestures*. Next, he would select a series of two or three fixed points, and practice moving his hand specifically from one point to another, then add a specific rhythm. These rhythmic patterns would then be used to practice a routine of apparently non-specific movements that he calls *open* gestures, which are looser and made within a wider range of motion. There is a third category of *descriptive gestures*, in which he uses his hands to illustrate certain things and shapes. He continues to practice these three types of gestures—with his safety always a main priority—so that he is ready to use them as he makes his action plans in his daily life. It is part of his way of being that he calls "living in the next movement."
>
> Later Ian and Brenda explained how they move together to de-emphasize Ian's limitations. It was fascinating to hear the details; what made their team-work extraordinary was the level of planning required to make the interaction seem more normal.

Studying Ian over decades, Jonathan has tried to understand his movements scientifically rather than as magic. Mark's approach, with exquisite control and analysis of movement in his own peri-personal space but in relation to a watching other, allows another dimension to the understanding of Ian's gestures. And these are even more remarkable when you consider that for Ian—unlike magicians—practice does not lead to skilled movement but just a greater repertoire of movements to retain and to reproduce through thought and planning.

Actors, academics, and astronauts, dancers, scientists, and magicians, are all fascinated to meet Ian. Each group learns much about movement and position sense from him, as we all can, but each finds aspects of how Ian has learned to move which have resonance for their own ideas and practice. His singular journey to regain mobility, and his extraordinary attention to the minutiae of action and reaction, parallels their own explorations in their own disciplines. It is just unfortunate that whereas the refinements to movement of a magician or dancer are rewarded, Ian's expertise passes unnoticed.

Shaun Gallagher, a philosopher who sees our selfhood as being embodied, in the world and socially realized, has only met Ian twice, in Chicago, for a few days during the gesture work:

> Yet I feel as if I have met Ian many more times, and in a sense I have. I keep bumping into him in my work as a philosopher; he appears frequently in my own papers, and also in the papers by other philosophers and neuroscientists that I read. I first heard about Ian from Jonathan when we met in 1992 in Cambridge. I had been working on the distinction between body image and body schema, and we reached some consensus that this distinction was relevant to Ian's way of moving. Jonathan and I wrote a paper about this, and later did a presentation at a conference on Merleau-Ponty. I still meet up with people who remember our presentation—not because of us, but because they remember Ian's amazing way of coping with the loss of proprioception. I will not count the number of conference and workshop presentations that I've done where I've talked about Ian—not only to audiences of philosophers, but to neuroscientists, physicians, physical therapists, sports scientists, and so on. Suffice it to say that since 1992 I estimate that, on average, it would be at least twice a year. Invariably, in follow-up discussions the majority of questions are about Ian and the fascinating details about his capacity to control movement without proprioception. In my responses I find myself, like Jonathan, returning to Ian the person—not just the experimental subject—and reassuring the audience that despite the challenge, Ian has a life and flourishes. This is one of the important lessons I've learned about humanizing the experimental subject, from Jonathan and from meeting Ian.

When Jonathan talks about Ian, whether he is there co-presenting or not, while there are always questions about the neuroscience, even hard-nosed, skeptical scientists are also interested in the day to day, mundane details of how Ian copes and how he is. Even scientists are as fascinated by the human details as the scientific data. Patrick Haggard made a similar reflection on his work with Ian:

> What have I learned? If you want to understand what a particular experience is like, then first-person testimony from people who live with that particular experience is

the best bet. The interesting thing is, most of us become rather self-indulgent, even a bit irritating, when we describe our experiences in a very first-person way. Ian doesn't; his first-person experience has an enormous scientific and medical value for the rest of us to learn from. His great gift is the open, generous, and pro-social way that he presents himself, and his own experiences. It's an interesting model of what it means to be human. I think Ian's approach confirms that we are at our best when we connect to others.

In one of Merleau-Ponty's last papers, he wrote:

Science manipulates things and gives up living in them.[6]

Arguably, the most powerful way to understand the world and ourselves is through science with its empirical and sometimes reductionist methods. But equally, an understanding of chronic neurological impairment is informed not only by empirical science, whether with high-tech imaging or string and sticky tape, but also by first-person accounts of what it is like to live with—and in—conditions long term, and through listening, questioning, and observing over months and years. We hope, in *Losing Touch*, that we have shown the need for and rewards of both approaches.

NOTES

Introduction

1. Bell, C. (1833). *The Hand; its Mechanism and Vital Endowments as Evincing Design*. Bridgewater Treatise. Reprinted in 1979 by The Pilgrims Press: Brentwood, UK. This book is an astounding exposition of proprioception and of neuroscience theory way before its time. *Pride and a Daily Marathon* (Cole J. 1991, 1995 Duckworth: London and then MIT Press: Cambridge, MA) was written, in part, as a dialogue with Bell.
2. It was first described by a New York neurologist, Herb Schaumburg, and his team: Sherman AB, Schaumberg HH, Ashbury AK. The acute sensory neuronopathy syndrome; a distinct clinical entity. *Ann Neurol* 1980;7:354–358.
3. Ian has destroyed all photos of himself from this time.
4. Rothwell JC, Traub MM, Day BL, Obeso JA, Thomas PK, Marsden CD. Manual motor performance in a deafferented man. *Brain* 1982;105:515–542.
5. In contrast Ian did have normal perceptions to clinical tests of pain and temperature, suggesting intact A-delta and C sensory nerve function. Jonathan and Haider wondered if, for the first time ever, they could record cortical potentials relayed through A-delta fibers from Ian. Usually any late activity is obscured by the larger faster A-beta-mediated wave. They also knew that the electrical shocks through the skin to stimulate A-delta fibers would be painful. Ian, after a discussion, was happy to have a go, though Jonathan did the experiment on himself first to make sure. It was painful, but tolerable. Ian's threshold for feeling the shock applied to a nerve at the wrist was 15 mA, five times normal. At high stimulus intensities, 39 mA, and with a longer duration of stimulus than used normally, 400 µs, a cortical potential was recorded with a latency of 84 ms from wrist to scalp, giving a velocity of 11.9 m/s, well in the range of A-delta sensory nerves. The peripheral nerve tests and cortical potentials all supported Ian's reports of him having a complete loss of those nerves underpinning the sensations of touch and movement/position sense, but having normal movement or motor nerves and intact smaller sensory nerves. Cole JD, Katifi HA. Evoked potentials in a man with a complete large fibre sensory neuropathy below the neck. *Electroenceph Clin Neurophysiol* 1991;80:103–107.
6. Cole JD, Sedgwick EM. The perceptions of force and of movement in a man without large myelinated sensory afferents below the neck. *J Physiol* 1992;449:503–515.
7. Cole JD, Merton LW, Barrett G, Treede R-D, Katifi H. Evoked potentials in a deafferented subject. *Can J Physiol Pharmacol* 1995;73:234–245.
8. Next Ian was asked to *imagine* moving his thumb. When control subjects did this they could not produce any reduction in threshold for a TMS-induced twitch. In contrast when Ian only imagined moving the thumb reduced thresholds were found for TMS-induced twitch in the thumb muscles alone. Even imagining led to some motor cortex change. And when during these experiments some sham stimuli and some real ones

were used, with Ian watching, he was very indignant when an imagined intention summed with a TMS-induced current to produce a twitch. "I did not do that!" he said, knowing the difference between him intending a movement and imagining the same thing. This result was published in the 1995 paper and then, years later, the experiment was repeated with Ian and Ginette Lizotte, a Québécois woman with a similar condition, in John Rothwell's lab in Queen Square. Ian's results were the same, but interestingly Ginette could not focus her intention in this way on a single muscle or movement at all. To work at Queen Square, Jonathan drove to Ian's house, picked him up, drove into the center of London, dropped Ian at the lab, parked the car some way away, and then went back to assist with the experiment. The journey took just under 3 hours. Then, after a coffee and a chat, the experiment took 15 minutes, after which Ian and Jonathan drove back. They even did it twice, because the first time John forgot to hit the "save" button!

9. Ian meant it as a short-hand for the way in which people with disability feel they must prove themselves and how the press follows them eagerly. His invention of the term preceded the several one-legged men and women who have now climbed Everest.

10. Much of the science with which Ian has assisted is not detailed since, excellent though it was, it did not have relevance for Ian's development as a neuroscience participant or did not alter the way he viewed his condition. These include several visits to the Max Planck Institute in Munich under Professor Prinz, and working with Simone Shultz-Bosbach, Gisa Aschersleben, and Prisca Stenneken. Much time there was spent pursuing the way in which Ian times action (taps) without peripheral feedback. See: Drewing K, Stenneken P, Cole J, Prinz W, Aschersleben G. Timing of bimanual movements and deafferentation: implications for the role of sensory movement effects. *Exp Brain Res* 2004;15850–57 and Stenneken P, Prinz W, Cole J, Paillard J, Aschersleben G. The effect of sensory feedback on the timing of movements: evidence from deafferented patients. *Brain Res* 2006:1084:123–131.The other main experiment was on the way in which Ian and Ginette Lizotte make judgments about the expectations of another when that person picks up an unknown weight. The experiments were able to show that Ian and Ginette were as accurate as controls in assessing the actual weights picked up, but that they had deficits in recognizing the other's *expectation* of the weights picked up. See: Bosbach S, Cole J, Prinz W, Knoblich G. Inferring another's expectation from action: the role of peripheral sensation. *Nat Neurosci* 2005;8:1295–1297.This was the subject of another article: Narain C. Thinking outside the box. *Nat Rev Neurosci* 2005;6:821.

11. Ian was never keen on the title of the TV documentary, "The Man Who Lost His Body," though he accepted its dramatic utility. He had after all not really lost his body, he just did not know where it was without looking. Yet it was lost to his unconscious control and certainly touch and proprioception were gone forever. In work with Ian many people have focused on his proprioceptive deficit since it is so extraordinary and since its effects on movement are so dramatic (though so well disguised by Ian most of the time). The title of the present account, *Losing Touch: a Man Without His Body*, is used to emphasize Ian's literal loss of touch but also to imply a loss of touch generally with the body. "Without" runs the same risks of interpretation as "lost." But it is meant in the sense of "not having or making use of normally, as being outside, or not accompanied by in a normal manner." In the end it is not surprising that such an unusual sensory impairment is difficult to capture in a short phrase, but it is hoped that this title balances catchiness with insight.

12. Corkin S (2013). *Permanent Present Tense*. Allen Lane: London.

Chapter 1

1. In English "monster" has freakish or ugly negative overtones, but in French it can be used for someone with outstanding gifts.
2. His brothers did soon work out that if, when he was standing or walking, they threw a towel over Ian's feet so he could not see them then he would fall over, and they used this as a threat and a party trick.
3. Though, for Ian, even sitting is a task. He describes how in a secure chair he can place his body and know it will not move, though it may slowly slump, "like a sack of potatoes." Then he can relax a bit and start to gesture and chat more freely.
4. He loves hanging out in a café, watching the world go by, or having a beer and maybe a meal, just sitting around observing others for a change.
5. When doing experiments Jonathan will, where possible, take Ian to the place the day before so Ian can familiarize himself with the layout and work out his moves.
6. When Jonathan stayed with Ian he used to run up the hills. Once, soon after he set off, he saw a small figure way in the distance above. Eventually Jonathan caught him and had a chat. He was an old schoolteacher who had retired to where he had started out, in Sedburgh. Well into his 70s, he still walked the hills each day. In his younger days he was an international runner. Initially he ran middle distances, 880 yards up to 3 miles. But, after losing a lung in the war, he had had to drop down to 440 yards since he did not have as much puff.
7. Robert Murphy, who became immobile late in life, wrote of how, "a quadriplegic's body can no longer speak a 'silent language' ... the thinking activity can no longer be dissolved into motion, and the mind can no longer be lost in an internal dialogue with physical movement." Murphy R (1987). *The Body Silent*. Henry Holt: New York. A consideration of the pleasure coming from movement is to be found in: Cole JD, Montero B. Affective proprioception. *Janus Head* 2006;9:299–320.
8. Jonathan mentioned Ian's memory for buildings and access to Linda. "It's like that for me with cakes," she replied.

Chapter 2

1. Standing is something we take for granted, and yet it is an inherently unstable process. Martin Lackie and colleagues in the University of Birmingham talk of the body acting as in inverted pendulum when standing, with its weight at the top and a need to balance the whole time, which is usually unconscious. With ultrasound one can see the calf muscles constantly moving when we stand as we adjust to small changes in posture and weight distribution. [See Loram ID, Golle H, Lakie M, Gawthrop PJ. Human control of an inverted pendulum: is continuous control necessary? Is intermittent control effective? Is intermittent control physiological? *J Physiol* 2011;589:307–324.]
2. Amazingly adept though he is, one of the main limitations on Ian's ability to move is speed of action. He cannot run because, in part, he needs time to work out all the various aspects of the movement.
3. Ballet and other dancers often "spot," i.e. look at fixed positions on a wall or floor, so they can orientate themselves in relation to the external world during fast spins and lifts. People who live from wheelchairs do the same in order to keep their head and body upright when they cannot feel below the neck. Ian also does this, gaining clues about his overall body position and uprightness from spots he sees in his environment.

4. Next time you use stairs in a public building have a look. Most times the hand rail starts at the first step or higher, when it really should start before (or after) the steps have finished, giving someone support as they get on or off the stairs.

5. Ian has developed claustrophobia which for the most part he manages, though it has stopped any thoughts of functional imaging experiments in which subjects have to lie in small, enveloping tunnels.

6. In unpublished work from Mike Land's lab at the University of Sussex Ian's eye movements and gait were monitored as he walked through the university building and then out into the campus. The rapidity and complexity of his gaze was far more detailed than that of control subjects. When he walked down an office corridor his eyes shot sideways every few steps. On analyzing this we were puzzled until we realized he was checking that each door was shut and that no one was about to come out unexpectedly and balk him.

7. Ian has a catalogue of neuroscientists with "idiosyncratic" driving styles. In Quebec, with the late Jacques Paillard, waiting at a large intersection Jacques got bored: "Shall we go now?" Ian replied, "No, Jacques, I would wait for the red light to change." Jean Blouin used to collect Ian and Jonathan from their bed and breakfast accommodation in Le Vieux Port in Marseilles to take them to the lab. But Jean only knew the route to his place of work from his own flat, so he always drove back to his place first, even when retracing his route meant going the wrong way down one way streets in the middle of Marseille at rush hour. How respiratory physiologist Abe Guz survived driving for years through London is a complete mystery and reflects on everyone else's ability to get out of his way.

8. The work on Ian has not been published. One review of his work is Mittelstaedt H. Somatic graviception. *Biol Psychol* 1996;42:53–74. A précis follows:

Psychophysical experiments, as performed by Ian, show that the perception of posture in the body in its horizontal axis is to a large degree affected by two hitherto unknown graviceptor systems in the human trunk. In studies involving the tilt table and the horizontal platform of the rotating centrifuge, subjects were asked to return themselves to when they felt horizontal, while in the dark. Where that horizontal axis was felt differed between control subjects and those with various neurological impairments. Control subjects set the centrifuge axis on average at 22–28 cm behind, i.e. more towards the body, than the inner ear's balance and orientation organ, while those with neurological loss of sensation from the body and leg set it further back, 45–55 cm.

This suggests that the receptors underpinning this perception should be situated near the last ribs. Further experiments on paraplegic patients lead to the conclusion that gravity perception from the body is mediated by two distinctly localized inputs, the first entering the spinal cord at the eleventh thoracic segment, and the second reaching the brain cranial of the sixth cervical segment, presumably via the phrenic or vagus nerves. (These are two so-called cranial nerves which leave the brain quite high up in the brainstem area in the neck and then travel down into the body to innervate the lungs, heart, and guts.)

By doing a series of experiments on people with spinal cord injury at various levels, Mittelstaedt was able to show two effects, one in subjects with spinal cord injury at the eleventh thoracic vertebra and another in those with a level higher, at the sixth cervical or neck vertebra. The effect of the first input is abolished after bilateral removal of the kidneys, so proving that they affect gravity perception. Ian also showed this effect. He has not, of course, lost his kidneys, but has lost the large sensory nerves coming from them, so in turn his results suggest that the perception depends on large myelinated sensory nerves arising in the kidney itself. In contrast the second input was revealed by experiments on the centrifuge, which has the effect of shifting the inertial mass in the body, which may in turn be that of the blood in the large vessels. In the centrifuge experiments Ian behaved like the control subjects since his small nerves to the blood vessels of the abdomen and legs are intact. In comparison, subjects with high spinal cord lesions, who had lost small sensory nerves from the large blood vessels of the abdomen as well as legs formed a different population. The inertial forces involved in this dynamic Z-axis perception are measured by mechanoreceptors in the structures that mechanically support the large blood vessels.

9. In retrospect this was one of the first manifestations of Ian's claustrophobia.

10. Treede RD, Cole JD. Dissociated secondary hyperalgesia in a subject with a large-fibre sensory neuropathy. *Pain* 1993;53:169–74.

This work investigated what happens to the skin around an area of injury. Soon after, this area becomes more sensitive to touch, so-called hyperalgesia to mechanical (touch) stimuli. Two types of this secondary hyperalgesia have been found, one to light stroking touch and the second to punctate stimuli, as in when a pencil tip is touched to the skin. These two have different durations and sizes of area involved.

The experiments studied secondary hyperalgesia in Ian after the injection of 60 μg of capsaicin to produce temporary injury. Stroking with a cotton swab was not perceived anywhere on affected skin either before or after injection. Thus, there was no hyperalgesia to light touch. Capsaicin injection into the volar forearm evoked normal pain and flare. A von Frey probe exerting a force of 40 mN was perceived as sharp. The sensation of sharpness was more pronounced up to 2 cm outside the flare zone for at least 16 minutes following the injection (tested with a 200 mN von Frey probe). Thus, hyperalgesia to punctate stimuli developed as in control subjects. These data support the model that hyperalgesia to light touch (allodynia) is due to sensitization of central pain-signaling neurons to low-threshold mechanoreceptor input (A-beta fibers). In contrast, punctate hyperalgesia is likely to be due to sensitization to nociceptor input (A-delta or C fibers). Wittgenstein famously wrote, "I do not know I am in pain." Most people interpret this as meaning that the verb in the sentence is inappropriate, we do not "know" pain; we experience it at another more immersed, immediate level. But this experiment made Jonathan question whether Wittgenstein also doubted the pronoun. What does "I" mean when consumed by pain thus? Cole described it thus:

'The experimentally induced pain filled my world and it became difficult to localize precisely where it was. It was out there, though I was no longer sure quite what that meant. It filled my arm, my body and destroyed, for a short time, my sense of self in the sense of my awareness of my body and also in the sense of my memory of what was going on. We live with a perception of our bodies as a whole. Even when not attending to it I felt a presence of my body, say, of an arm or a leg. But with the pain I no longer thought in such terms. I had pain which took over completely so that localization was impossible. I no longer had a background idea of my hand or arm at all; the pain removed my feeling of being in a body; I just had and was pain. Moreover, I could not think. I did not know I was in pain certainly, but, in addition, I no longer knew quite what "I" was; whatever that might be, it was a me-with-pain, no longer an "I," no longer a self-observing the world or even immersed in it. The pain was so consuming that the world, as an external place to calibrate myself in, and from, no longer presented itself and my sense of being a "me" was no longer valid either.'

Cole, J. *Still Lives* (2004; MIT Press: Cambridge, MA), pp. 7–8

Wittgenstein had his gall bladder removed without anesthetic. Turgenev was also conscious throughout his abdominal operation due to an anesthetic problem, though he may not have written about it. As the nineteenth-century writer Alphonse Daudet wrote, "Pain is normally the enemy of descriptive powers ... like passion [it] drives out language." Words came, "only when everything is over, when things have calmed down." (Daudet A. *In the Land of Pain*, edited and translated by Barnes J (2002) Jonathan Cape: London, p. v). (Daudet lived with excruciating destructive chronic pain as a result of syphilis.) Cole describes how his severe pain reduced after a few minutes and that he could then begin to observe and analyze his sense of self: an "I" had returned, rejoining the others in the room, in the world. After 12 minutes or so the pain was gone and he could joke about the "minor irritation" Ian was about to enjoy. Ian did the experiment. Some experiments, they agreed, are more fun than others.One difference between Ian and Cole was in the localization of the pain. Ian remembers, "I knew where the pain was, but if someone had moved my arm around I would not have known where that was." In other words he knew that the pain was in his forearm, but he had no awareness of where that arm was. He had a map of pain and temperature on his body, but no map of where his body was in space, an extraordinary idea. (Tony Marcel first drew Cole's attention to this.)

11. "The Civil Service was very good. I went to Human Relations and asked for time off for research to look at how I move in Germany. They gave me paid leave; they never understood it so they thought they had better not stop it."

12. Ian is probably being a little unfair. Over the years, Cole has met Rolf-Detlef at meetings and he always asks after Ian, even 20 years later.

13. Academics often like to claim that science is done in a Popperian way, confirming or refuting a prior hypothesis. But often scientists are following educated hunches. At one meeting Cole listened as someone presented his results and then announced that the results confirmed his prior hypothesis, mainly because they came up with the hypothesis after he had done the experiment. Everyone cheered.

14. This is not to say that walking is normal for Ian, see *Pride and a Daily Marathon*, pp. 126ff.

15. Many neuroscience experiments ended up with string and sticky tape when Ian was involved. Initially Ian was surprised at how amateurish this appeared. Slowly he realized that the scientists were usually doing new things and stressing both his and their abilities.

16. Charles Bell wrote in 1833 of how the accomplishment of any small movement actually involves the automatic contraction of many muscles in the body. [Bell C (1833). *The Hand; its Mechanism and Vital Endowments as Evincing Design*. Bridgewater Treatise. Reprinted in 1979 by The Pilgrims Press: Brentwood, UK.]

17. The aim of the experiment was actually to investigate end-point versus amplitude errors. When moving between positions, one theory suggests that the accuracy of reaching to a position depends on knowing where one starts from. When Ian moved from, say, positions one to three he might have overshot; then, under an amplitude model, this overshoot would be expected to affect the accuracy of the next reach, and so on. The alternative theory, the end-point model, suggests that we can reach many positions independent of starting position by computing the end positions independent of where we are to start with. Ian performed mainly according to an amplitude model, as was anticipated, but was more accurate for positions one and nine, as he had said, or imagined what those were, and for the mid position. This work has not yet been published, in part because a similar experiment, though arguably less refined, has been published

from work with Ginette Lizotte and Ian from Canada. The record delay between experiment and paper stands at 14 years and counting, for two important pieces of work.

18. Matthews' book, *Mammalian Muscle Receptors and their Central Actions*, published in 1982, summarized work in the field and was 400 pages long. One summer, somewhat sadly in retrospect, Cole read it from cover to cover. Peter Matthews was a tall, lean man who cycled everywhere wearing a beret. During lectures, when not gesturing, he would fold his arms up beside him like a heron.

Chapter 3

1. You are not aware of the weight of your limbs or body; they are a given. Similarly you do not feel twice as much weight going through one leg when standing on it compared with two legs. Ian, though not able to feel weight or force, had to be acutely aware of its consequences and control for them. But when under increased gravitational force, say in a 2g centrifuge or parabolic flight, then you do become very aware of how heavy you feel when standing on one leg.

2. Miall RC, Cole JD. Evidence for stronger visuo-motor than visuo-proprioceptive conflict during mirror drawing performed by a deafferented subject and control subjects. *Exp Brain Res* 2007;176:432–439. There is some evidence from experiments on prism adaptation that Ginette can form these programs in other circumstances.

3. Bell, C. (1833). *The Hand; its Mechanism and Vital Endowments as Evincing Design*. Bridgewater Treatise, p. 199. Reprinted in 1979 by The Pilgrims Press: Brentwood, UK.

4. Subsequently we published the more formal tests of Ginette's abilities to perceive weights. Fleury M, Bard C, Teasdale N, Paillard J, Cole J D, Lajoie Y, Lamarre Y. Weight judgement: the discrimination capacity of a deafferented subject. *Brain* 1995;118:1149–1156. More complex experiments on the relation between central and peripheral signals in the judgment of weight were subsequently performed with Richard Fitzpatrick (see Luu BL, Day BL, Cole JD, Fitzpatrick RC. The fusimotor and reafferent origin of the sense of force and weight. *J Physiol* 2011;589:3135–3147).

5. They were met by Jean-Louis Vercher and driven to their bed and breakfast, a charming small pension on Le Vieux Port; from their windows they looked out on the ships, shops, smugglers, and thieves alleged to control that bit of the Med. They arrived on a Sunday, traditionally Demonstration Day in France. This was a classic; taxi drivers versus police. Ian watched from his front window as Marseille's finest marched round, just below the hotel. They were being stopped by a row of riot police, all in their Sunday best; riot shields, truncheons, helmets, and visors. Protests were shouted and gesticulated on the one side and, 50 m away, truncheons were banged against riot shields. Then, in between the two, Ian saw this skinny runner saunter between the two groups, the effect heightened by a pair of Union Jack shorts. By the time Jonathan got back they had dispersed, and Ian never found out what they were protesting about.

6. Blouin J, Gauthier G M, Vercher J-L, Cole J. The relative contribution of retinal and extra-retinal signals in determining the accuracy of reaching movements in normal subjects and a deafferented patient. *Exp Brain Res* 1996;109:148–153.

7. Vercher J-L, Gauthier G M, Guedon O, Blouin J, Cole J, Lamarre Y. Self-moved target eye tracking in control and deafferented subjects: roles of arm motor command and proprioception in arm eye coordination. *J Neurophysiol* 1997;76:1133–1144.Vercher J-L, Gauthier G, Cole J, Blouin J. Role of arm proprioception in calibrating the arm-eye temporal coordination. *Neurosci Lett* 1997;237:1–4.

8. Alas, this is one of the more important pieces of work that has never been published.
9. Blue Peter is a TV program for children in the UK. Among other things it showed children how to make things with "sticky back plastic" and string, and so is a synonym for a Heath Robinson contraption.

Chapter 4

1. Linda was kind enough to have a long talk with Jonathan, but in the end wanted her thoughts to remain unpublished. Ian too has discussed this, but did not want to trawl over things again.
2. Stephen Duckworth was interviewed in *Still Lives*, in the chapter "Disability Matters." He is now working in a high-up position advising the UK government.
3. In 2006 Jonathan chaired the world conference in Edinburgh for his medical specialty. Towards its end, a friend volunteered "Great conference," Jonathan asked about the best bit. His friend thought for a moment before replying, "The coffee."
4. As time went by, however, Mike became more interested. A few years later he used to sit with Ian in front of clients and ask how the filming with the BBC was going (see Chapter 6).
5. As work developed Ian was in London more regularly and always booked a taxi in advance to avoid queuing. Once, when taking his mother, he booked a taxi to meet the train as usual, and she was so impressed. He loved showing off to her.
6. They asked Ian to audit their hotels for staff holidays. He turned one down, on an island, because he could not get on the ferry.
7. Fortunately they are now friends. Once, when discussing with Jonathan their time together, Linda paused and said, "He is the bravest man I have ever met. I am in awe of him, always have been and always will be. Who wouldn't be?"

Chapter 5

1. Bradby D, Delgado MM (ed.) (2002). "Playful understanding": an interview with David Bennent. *The Paris Jigsaw: Internationalism and the City's Stages*, pp. 55–56. Manchester University Press: Manchester.
2. Ian's portrayal occurred just over half way through the play. Other vignettes were of cortical stimulation to map areas of the brain before epilepsy surgery, perseverant behavior with frontal lobe lesions, autism, memory loss, visual agnosia, various forms of neglect, Tourette's, musical epilepsy, aphasia, and blindsight. Tourette's syndrome, with uncontrollable spitting, tics, and swearing, is a tremendously theatrical, almost operatic, disease. In contrast, there were some beautiful, muted, internalized dramas. In one, Yoshi Oida portrayed a man hearing, as the audience did, some beautiful classical music. He, like us, was not sure where it was coming from; maybe the radio, maybe outside the room, maybe wherever. He was torn between enjoying it and worrying about its origin. A doctor came along to explain that the music he heard was inside his head and was a form of epilepsy. This was a comfort to know, but then some pills quietened down the epileptic discharge and abolished the music; recovery and regret combined. Yoshi portrayed all this with few words, a performance of simple beauty to match Sacks' prose and observation. Yoshi also portrayed the final scene, a man with hemi-neglect. He is asked to shave in a mirror and shaves one side of his face. Then he is

shown a recording of his shave. It becomes clear what he has done, and that the mirror side and the video side of the face are different. His fragile sense of self, cobbled together in the face of such a condition, dissolves. It is interesting that in several of the vignettes people with neglect are confronted with their condition. Jonathan was always taught that this just confuses and threatens the person, since they cannot assimilate this with their elaborate mental delusions and constructions designed to maintain a semblance of cohesion to their sense of self. Jonathan sat at the back with a friend of Oliver's who had Tourette's syndrome and who had helped with that vignette. During the performance, he had to go out every so often to give vent to his tics and swearing before coming back in, calmer, to watch the show again. When the Tourette vignette was on, the whole place was alive and he was able to be a bit more forthcoming with his appreciation, and his tics. At Bouffes du Nord Maurice Benichou, who had joined the company later, performed the Tourette's scene. It is the most boisterous part of the play and one in which he addresses the audience more directly. Ever a showman, he was swearing and spitting over the front seats and the whole place was going along with his excess. Maurice turned to go off, thought for a moment, and then turned back. "It's no fun to be like this all the time, you know." Laughing and whooping one moment, the next everyone stopped and drew breath.

3. After performances Peter would do question and answer sessions with the audience. Many questions were about the writing of the play, and technical and medical questions, while others were about Peter himself and his career. But at one session a woman stood up, rather hot under the collar. "Why are there no women on stage?" [The cast was four male actors.] Peter, who has spent his career trying to rid people of seeing things literally, looked pained. "But there are women; they are just played by men." The feminist was flummoxed and fortunately sat down quietly.

4. The play was then revived a couple of years later with Bruce Myers portraying Ian. Jonathan and Ian went to London to give him some tips before it opened. More recently the play was revived by the Central Drama School at the Guildhall in London. How would it do without the Brook stardust? In fact the students and director were brilliant. Brook's production was spare and spaced, with four actors and a single musician, whereas this was much larger ensemble piece, with 20 or so in the cast on the stage the whole time. Jonathan was asked to assist with the accuracy of the neurological portrayals, not just Ian's. Being introduced to the students as someone involved in the original production he had rarely felt as old. Ian's vignette finished the show and was performed by a female actor. She was excellent in her aping of Ian's movements and in her balance between illness and hope.

Chapter 6

1. There are a number of clinical papers concerned with documenting sensory neuronopathy syndrome caused by autoimmune disease or drugs given for some cancers. Two good recent ones, detailing diagnosis and management are: Camdessanche J-P, Jousserand G, Ferraud K,Vial C, Petiot P, Honnorat J, Antoine J-C. The pattern and diagnostic criteria of sensory neuronopathy: a case–control study. *Brain* 2009;132:1723–1733 and Sheikh SI, Amato A A. The dorsal root ganglion under attack: the acquired sensory ganglionopathies. *Pract Neurol* 2010;10:326–334. These papers are excellent clinical accounts, but the patients in these papers do not appear to have engaged with the neuroscience in terms of the experience of living with severe sensory loss.

2. Ian was kind, and did not go on to other aspects of walking with Charles. For though Ian walks, the constraints he lives with make this a very different action. He cannot put his weight on a bent leg in case the knees gives way, so he always lands on a braced leg. Neither can he rise up onto his toes since the ankles might give way. So he lands on the heels, like a duck on water, and takes off from the back of the foot. To avoid scuffing the foot on the floor at that leg goes forward, he abducts the hip to turn the foot outwards, making his gait a little Chaplinesque. And to see what is happening to his limbs, his head is tilted forward, so he balances this by having his arms not only out for balance but also a little back. He walks but in his way. Having said this, his gait looks closer to normal than it is. But it is dependent on Ian's attention. So, Jonathan can tell how tired he is by how clean his walking is.

3. Neither Charles nor Ian could propel themselves by gripping the wheels of the chair with the hands, like paraplegics. They could not feel the wheels nor look at each wheel in turn to propel themselves easily. Interestingly, Ginette, in a wheelchair from early on, has mastered this.

4. On a train trip from London, Jonathan once watched Ian get off at a station with a low platform. Ian had to make a similar "ballistic" drop of 6 inches or so from train to platform. No one watching would have seen saw anything odd, but for less than a second he was descending with little control and Jonathan was very concerned. Afterwards Ian agreed it had been hairy.

5. They left Pittsburgh wondering whether Charles would manage to move much better. He was much older so that learning to move again must be so much harder. Ian was not sure either that Charles was prepared for the almost obsessive dedication to movement that was required.

6. At this point his dreams of becoming an astronaut faded. Chris Rawlence, in contrast, had never been keen on space, likening a shuttle mission to a 2-week holiday stuck inside a caravan.

7. The engineers had programmed a slight grasp into the hands with a servo motor, so once he had put the fingers to the egg, the robot took over to produce the right amount of grip. Without feedback of applied force, and with an isometric grip required for the egg, since it would have broken if gripped even a little, the task would otherwise be difficult for anyone.

8. Subsequently, virtual reality research has shown the same thing, as has the elegant work of Olaf Blanke and Henrik Ehrsson. A short letter describing the phenomenon was published by Jonathan, Oliver, and Ian: Cole J, Sacks O, Waterman I. On the immunity principle: a view from a robot. *Trends Cogn Sci* 2000;4:167. See also Sacks O (2012). *Hallucinations*. Knopf: New York and Picador: London.

9. BBC *Horizon*. Rosetta Pictures, director Chris Rawlence, producer Emma Crichton-Miller, camera Chris Morphet.

10. "Suffering is nothing. It's all a matter of preventing those you love from suffering." (Daudet A. *In the Land of Pain*, edited and translated by Barnes J (2002) Jonathan Cape).

11. This showed that he still has some automatic compensatory movements. Another example is the waiter's tray illusion. When we are carrying drinks on a tray, if someone takes a drink then we cannot help but raise the tray a little afterwards. But if we take the drink off ourselves the tray does not rise. Ian shows this as well.

12. Degas often painted and sculpted dancers during a move in mid-position. To freeze that in a photo was easy; to hold it in real life near impossible.

13. After they met Jonathan had asked Marsha, on her next mission, to do a simple experiment if she had time. She came back with some film of astronauts floating, eyes shut and

arms out-stretched. On her command they had to move one hand to touch a finger on the other. Some found it really difficult to touch finger to finger precisely, unless they moved the target hand a little too, to reset the body's awareness of itself.

14. It is not often on television that one sees an actual experiment being performed, rather than a reproduction.

15. Again they recorded as they experimented in real time. Unfortunately these results have not yet been published.

16. But not all the people contacting us were new or ill. One unexpected viewer was the mother of Ian's girlfriend at the time of his original illness. When ill, and at a low ebb, Ian had broken things off with her. Now, nearly 30 years later she had a grown family and was divorced. She and Ian met and got together for a short, intense affair.

Chapter 7

1. See http://www.age-of-the-sage.org/scientist/stephen_hawking_zero-gravity.html.

2. Jonathan ran into a serious problem, mild asthma, which was "an absolute contraindication to flying the KC135." To prove his fitness he underwent a histamine challenge test. In this test histamine, a potent initiator of asthma, is squirted down into the lungs in ever-increasing doses until the subject starts wheezing seriously. Jonathan passed this without any wheeze or other signs of asthma. Neither the doctor, nor NASA, asked themselves whether Jonathan, himself a doctor, might have known which antihistamine drug to take!

3. Russian cosmonauts were put up here too. There was a rumor that, unaccustomed to the luxury, they all moved into one apartment and let out the others, sharing the profits.

4. Paul never left Ian's side and was fully equipped to assist him if necessary.

5. In the build-up Jim and Paul had explained that everyone vomited and that it was not a problem. They told of one group they had taken up. Wanting naïve controls with no drugs on board, they had recruited from a Southern Bible College. As the plane took off they all started singing hymns. The experiment involved spinning in a rotating chair as gravity changed. Each student was brought up to the chair, spun and then started vomiting. They were then laid on the floor at the back of the plane with the others. At the end of the flight there was a lot of hosing down to do. Having finished this anecdote, Jim said, matter-of-factly, that he had never been sick and Paul piped up that he hadn't either. OK, Jonathan thought, he would not be sick either, for Britain and for British physiology.

6. Jonathan is sympathetic to phenomenological and enactive accounts which disagree with reductionist views of the self as being in the brain and the mind, arguing instead that we—our minds and body—are one, and that our consciousness is in the self and the body and the world. However, during zero gravity he did feel that he, himself, was looking out from the head and down at his body with an altered perspective and relation.

7. They had talked with an astronaut who had told of this odd upside-down perception. He had said that having experienced it in space aboard the Space Shuttle he could now imagine his way into seeing the floor inverted as the ceiling when back on Earth. Having had the same experience himself, albeit fleetingly, Jonathan can now imagine the same thing. Our imagination seems to an extent to be bound by our experience.

8. Although a prosthetic arm may feel heavy, even when it is lighter than a real arm.

9. Jonathan wrote an article for the Physiological Society's newsletter about flying on the KC135 and they reprinted the photo. Soon after, a lady from Wellcome Trust, who had kindly given supported the travel to America, rang Jonathan to ask if he would write something for them. Then she asked sheepishly, "And can we use the photo?" Cole J. Pulling G's aboard the Vomit Comet: physiology in weightlessness. *Physiol News* 2000;38:10–12. Cole J. Braving the Vomit Comet. *Wellcome News* 2000;23:24.

10. Jonathan was reluctant to discuss this with Jim, thinking he was over-interpreting. But Jim had noticed the same and has done experiments on it. He found that when one counts time to estimate it, then there is no difference in zero, 1 or 1.8g. But, they agreed, that time passing as one goes about one's business is very differently perceived than during a count when one's attention is on time alone.

Chapter 8

1. This was the time he did not phone Jonathan, knowing that Jonathan would have been torn between sorting him out medically and videoing his breakdown of movement.

2. At one point Brenda was concerned that she might have taken some things away from Ian that previously he could do, reducing his need for action and independence. She was also worried that she had come into his life and filled it with family, teenage boys, friends, and nursing her father. "Where did his quiet life go?" In truth she had improved his life a million-fold, allowing him to embrace and relish it anew.

3. This echoes Sir Ludwig Guttmann's approach at Stoke Mandeville after World War II. Asked what his aim was he once replied, "to turn my patients into tax payers."

4. Stephen Duckworth has gone from strength to strength and is now leading the UK government's disability training project.

5. When she slipped again and broke the other ankle they took the pins out of one leg and put new ones in the other, leaving her for a while without a good leg at all.

6. Except for research trips, Jonathan suggested, tongue in cheek.

Chapter 9

1. Cole J. (1991, 1995). *Pride and a Daily Marathon*. Duckworth: London, The MIT Press: Cambridge, MA, p. 148.

2. Thanks to the BBC for supporting one visit to Chicago and Wellcome Trust for supporting the subsequent one.

3. McNeill D. (2005). *Gesture and Thought*. Chicago University Press: Chicago, p. xi.

4. McNeill D. (1992). Hand and Mind. Chicago University Press: Chicago, pp. 75–104.

5. Vygotsky L. (1986). *Thought and Language*. The MIT Press: Cambridge, MA, p. 251.

6. McNeill D. (2005). *Gesture and Thought*. Chicago University Press: Chicago, p. 4.

7. McNeill D. (2005). *Gesture and Thought*. Chicago University Press: Chicago, pp. 99–101.

8. McNeill D. (2005). *Gesture and Thought*. Chicago University Press: Chicago, pp. 234ff.

9. Quaeghebeur L, Duncan S, Gallagher S, Cole J, & McNeill D. Aproprioception, gesture, and cognitive being, In: Müller C, Cienki A, Fricke E, Ladewig SH, McNeill D and Bressem J (eds) *Body–Language–Communication. An International Handbook on Multimodality in Human Interaction* (Handbook of Linguistics and Communication 38.2). De Gruyter Mouton: Berlin/Boston, pp 2026–2047.

10. Ian's view on this is the same as David's:

Is gesture for the speaker or the listener? Does it perform an internal function that aides lexical retrieval and/or boost fluency (in the speaker), or an external function of communicating information to the listener? I believe the distinction is simplistic or false. Each gesture is for both . . . The individual–social duality is inherent to gesture. A gesture is a bridge from one's social interaction to one's individual cognition . . . it depends on the presence (real or imagined) of the social other and yet is a dynamic element in the individual's cognition.

McNeill D (2005) *Gesture and Thought*.
Chicago University Press: Chicago, pp. 53–54

11. Cole J, Paillard J. (1995). Living without touch and peripheral information about body position and movement: studies with deafferented subjects. In: Bermudez J, Eilan N, Marcel A (eds) *The Body and the Self*, pp. 245–266. MIT Press: Cambridge, MA. (Reprinted in a paperback edition 1998.)

12. Gallagher S (2005). *How the Body Shapes the Mind*, Ch. 5. Oxford University Press: Oxford.

13. Others with a neuronopathy like Ian's remain ataxic, even years later. If Ian was not so from the beginning in gesture that would be remarkable. Alas no film of him from the early days exists.

14. Vygotsky was one of the first to stress the social origins of language and communication (see Note 5). This suggests that making the central command to gesture facilitates the finding of the right word, and that feedback from making the gesture itself is not necessary, at least proprioceptive feedback. This has parallels in an experiment with Ian performed by Jean-Louis Vercher in Marseille. Ian's ability to track a moving dot with his eyes quickly, without the movements degrading into catch-up saccadic eye movements, was improved if he moved the target dot himself with his hand rather than by machine. In other words, he can use, non-consciously, a motor program to move the arm to improve movement of the eyes.

Others with the condition all gesture, though only Ian and Jacqui McCoy, a subject with a similar condition to Ian who he met in New York (see Chapter 11), walk. Looking at their gestures, one also sees that, though compromised, the gestures are still individual. Charles' gestures are ataxic and close to his body, and unfurl slowly with his measured speech; Ginette's are somewhat similar. Ian and Jonathan recently met another member of the club, a Norwegian woman, with quite different gestures. She lives from a chair and is quite ataxic. Before her illness she worked her way round the world, with all those potential infections, and then fell ill once back in Norway, hardly germ central. She has red hair, big eyes, and so much vitality and energy it spills out through her movements. Safe—safe-ish at least—in her chair, her gestures and ataxia fuse into partially controlled performance. Ian has reduced spontaneous movements and controls everything; in contrast she lets it happen. Though she tucks her arms away when listening, to stop them moving, when talking she has so much gesture and movement it makes her appear more spontaneous and immersed in her body than Ian:

My gesture just came back, it just happened. In contrast to pick up a cup is difficult. Some gestures are easy and automatic. But if I am ill, then the gestures are less. In my chair and balanced, they are present. But if I have poor balance in the chair then I tell my hands not to move.

She, like Ian, spent over a year in rehab trying to walk:

Then I gave up I preferred to use my hands. Gestures came back after 2–3 months and were back to normal after 2 years or so. I did not think about it, they just came back.

Maybe Ian's gestures, like other movements, are more cognitive and controlled. Perhaps attribution of ownership of action differs between them, with Ian controlling everything and the Norwegian accepting ownership of a less controlled movement. Seeing Ian and her together was like watching Noh theater meet Keith Moon.

15. He has to go out of the house, down a steep short drive, and onto a pock-marked rough track, turning left past a muck heap from the stables down the road. After a short while the track bends right and up a short incline to the road, under trees from the wood. Overall it is around 300 meters; a small walk for humankind, but a massive achievement for Ian.

Chapter 10

1. Treede R-D, Cole JD. Dissociated secondary hyperalgesia in a subject with a large fibre sensory neuropathy. *Pain* 1993;53:169–174.

2. Though the peripheral conduction of C fibers is slow, once within the spinal cord it is roughly the same speed as that of A-deltas. This can be illustrated by sitting in an overly hot bath—you have two pains from putting your feet in the water, but a single feeling from your bottom.

3. Vallbo ÅB, Hagbarth K-E, Torebjörk HE, Wallin BG. Somatosensory, proprioceptive and sympathetic activity in human peripheral nerves. *Physiol Rev* 1979;59:919–957. This work could perhaps have attracted the interest of the Nobel Prize committee.

4. This paragraph has synthesized a huge amount of work, almost exclusively from Sweden, beginning with the pioneering work of Åke Vallbo and then of Johan Wessberg, Roland Johannson and Magnus Nordin, among others. See: Nordin M. Low-threshold mechanoreceptive and nociceptive units with unmyelinated (C) fibres in the human supraorbital nerve. *J Physiol* 1990;426:229–240. Olausson H, Wessberg J, Morrison I, McGlone F, Vallbo Å. The neurophysiology of unmyelinated tactile afferents. *Neurosci Biobehav Rev* 2010;34:185–191. Wessberg J, Olausson H, Fernström KW, Vallbo ÅB. Receptive field properties of unmyelinated tactile afferents in the human skin. *J Neurophysiol* 2003;89:1567–1575. Morrison I, Löken LS, Olausson H. The skin as a social organ. *Exp Brain Res* 2010;204:305–314.

5. Olausson H, Lamarre Y, Backlund H, Morin C, Wallin BG, Starck G, Ekholm S, Strigo I, Worsley K, Vallbo ÅB, Bushnell MC. Unmyelinated tactile afferents signal touch and project to insular cortex. *Nat Neurosci* 2002;5:900–904. Francis McGlone and Jonathan also studied Ian in the functional MRI scanner at Nottingham around this time, but unfortunately they ran into technical problems with their first attempt and were working on those when Håkan Olausson's beautiful work was published.

6. The frequency and importance of CT afferents remains a matter of some controversy. In some micro-neurography recordings, from the legs mainly, CT afferents have proved more difficult to record. See: Serra J, Campero M, Ochoa J, Bostock H. Activity-dependent slowing of conduction differentiates functional subtypes of C fibres innervating human skin. *J Physiol* 1999;515:799–811.

7. Our hotel was being renovated and breakfast had been moved to the top floor. It was early December and we sat looking out over the city which was covered by low, dark cloud. We started joking that for the dour Swedes this would be considered nice weather. Later in the day we went outside between labs. I was wheeling Ian, with Francis and Håkan walking beside. By now it was sleeting. Francis muttered, "It's turned out nice." Ian replied, "Yes, it could have gone either way." Håkan looked completely mystified, as usual, by his British guests.

8. It was also found that the other pain pathway, via A-delta fibers, which projects to cortical areas S1 and S2, inhibited CT afferent areas. Caetano G, Olausson H, Cole J, Jousmaki V, Hari R. Cortical responses to A delta-fiber stimulation: magnetoencephalographic recordings in a subject lacking large myelinated afferents. *Cereb Cortex* 2010;20:1898–1903.

     These experiments were in Riita Hari's lab in Helsinki. At the end of the experiments we wanted to look round the center of Helsinki and found a cab. We had been going a few minutes when, stopped at a red light, there was a sudden crash. The driver asked what had happened and I suggested that the lorry driver just moving away had hit our backside. Incensed, our man set off after the lorry. But, this being Helsinki, he pursued at the speed limit of 30 km/h. So we now enjoyed a slow car chase through the center of Helsinki until our driver could overtake and pull over in front of the lorry driver. Our man got out and a suitably frank exchange of views took place. A crowd assembled and the police were called. We were enjoying the spectacle too, until we realized he had kept the meter running and we were paying to watch. We interrupted the argument, paid our bill, and went the rest of the way on foot.

9. That some of these results might be the result of long-term plasticity is a concern, though Ginette's activations were similar enough to controls to make this unlikely.

10. Sherrington CS (1900). Cutaneous sensation. In: Schäfer EA (ed.) *Text-book of Physiology*, pp. 920–1001. Pentland: Edinburgh.

11. Foster RG, Provencio I, Hudson D, Fiske S, De Grip W, Menaker M. Circadian photoreception in the retinally degenerate mouse (rd/rd). *J Comp Physiol A* 1991;169:39–50.

12. Interestingly Ian does not feel the distinct perception of "wet" when he puts his hand in water. He feels what he describes as a "cold sensation enhanced because, say, I know the cat is wet." "Wet" is an elaborated perception rather than a peripherally originating sensation, a "touch blend," at least in part dependent on inputs through A-beta fibers, though one would imagine smaller fibers are involved too.

13. Some people with spinal cord injury report feeling touch on their insentient unfelt numb legs when they see their legs being touched, and this is presumably a form of multisensory integration when seen touch becomes felt touch. (See Cole J (2004) *Still Lives*. The MIT Press: Cambridge, MA.)

14. Large myelinated and C fibers are both found with rich interconnections within the skin of the glans of the penis and the clitoris, which is unlike the skin anywhere else. It is also likely that the receptive properties of the nerve endings change between the flaccid and erect states as the cutaneous receptors change their orientation and shape as the penis or clitoris becomes erect. Ian's experience suggests that the C fibers may have a similar but greater contribution to pleasurable touch than elsewhere, but that they still act with A-beta neurons. C fibers alone may allow some feeling of pleasure, albeit reduced, but they do not appear sufficient for sensation to be normal. Without A-beta fiber function the temporary unpleasant sensation of touch over the glans shortly after orgasm may also be absent, suggesting that this special form of touch-allodynia also requires large sensory fibers. Since the cutaneous stimulation leading to pleasure before orgasm and discomfort after it may be the same stroking, factors within the spinal cord and brain are paramount in the sudden change in this feeling. In addition of course, contextual and interpersonal feelings are also of crucial importance, as Ian stresses. Francis McGlone, Rick Johnson, and Janniko Georgiadis are acknowledged for helpful discussions in this area.

15. Cole, J. Intimacy; views from impairment and neuroscience. *Emot Space Soc* 2014;13:87–94.

Chapter 11

1. This need for Ian's constant awareness of where his body is and how he moves it was considered conceptually by Gallagher and Cole. They suggested that Ian had lacked his unconscious body schema and partially replaced it by using his conscious body image to guide movement. Gallagher S, Cole J. Body image and body schema in a deafferented subject. *J Mind Behav* 1995;16:369–390.

2. When he was first admitted for rehabilitation the doctors thought Ian would always be in a wheelchair. In contrast, the physical therapists, who had little idea of the problem, saw a highly motived young man, and so presumed he would walk out and be independent.

3. In the Q&A session, Oliver asked if Ian dreamed whole or impaired. Ian answered that he was occasionally able-bodied and sometimes disabled.

4. In fact Ian's name very rarely appears on the papers as an author, which he is happy about. But there was one where he was. It may be a rather short observation, but the last two authors are special: Cole J, Sacks O, Waterman I. On the immunity principle: a view from a robot. *Trends Cogn Sci* 2000;4:167.

5. Guinea pigs are not pigs, nor from Guinea, and the term preceded the guinea coin. The "guinea" part could have derived from "Guineamen," sailing slavers' ships from the UK to Africa and then on to the Americas. The use of the term "pig" is easier. They look like small pigs and in the sixteenth century small and vaguely porcine creatures were often termed "pigs." The first use of the term "guinea pig" to describe a person was a name for inexperienced midshipmen on the sailing ships mentioned previously. It's present meaning, "subject of an experiment," has been traced to George Bernard Shaw, in *Quintessence of Ibsenism Now Completed* (1913):

   > The . . . folly which sees in the child nothing more than the vivisector sees in a guinea pig: something to experiment on with a view to rearranging the world.

   (Information from: http://www.phrases.org.uk/meanings/guinea-pig.html)

6. See, Firestein S (2012). *Ignorance*. Oxford University Press: New York and Oxford. Stuart Firestein explores how science is guided by what he calls ignorance but which is really curiosity about how things work.

7. E-mails from David McNeill, August 27 and September 9, 2013 (reproduced with permission). In a further email Jonathan mentioned to David that he found his theory of how gesture and language are one to contain a beauty one sees all too rarely in science. David replied:

   > It's always interested me that physicists see beauty and truth connected. Psychologists, at least the American variety, don't. For them, the first question is epistemological: How do you know? There is a skepticism instilled in them as students. The most admired departments reek of it the most. They don't seem to see the beauty of a whole that incorporates separate parts in its own construction, a kind of self-reference—and how they are not parts as a result. This is one kind of beauty and, I think, of truth. Of all the conglomerates the beautiful one is likely to be true. I've also often wondered though if the beauty–truth connection is more than skin deep (to work the metaphor to death). If we think of beauty as some quality of wholes, and that truth is also, there may be a deeper connection. All this is the flat opposite of reductionist truth, where what is true is finding the elements and how they combine; the whole is a product then, not a truth. Here, beauty lies in the cleverness of the combinations of parts, and maybe in the choice of parts as well. The two beauties simply don't mesh.

8. As they left the lab Brenda asked Ian if he was really that annoyed. The answer was yes, though it was expressed more earthily than that.

9. Mechsner F, Stenneken P, Cole J, Aschersleben G, Prinz W. Bimanual circling in de-afferented patients: evidence for a role of visual forward models. *J Neuropsychol* 2007;1:259–282.

10. *Financial Times*, June 13, 2014.

11. From Bell C (1833). *The Hand; its Mechanism and Vital Endowments as Evincing Design.* Bridgewater Treatise. Reprinted in 1979 by The Pilgrims Press: Brentwood, UK.

12. During the making of one TV series, Oliver and the film crew wandered round the Pacific as well as the USA and the UK. Jonathan was talking to the sound man, who said that during that time Oliver had never spoken to him, and added that he thought he only had time for the director. Jonathan knew this was not so and said that Oliver was shy and found small talk difficult. What was the sound man interested in? He said he was just researching a program on the outdoor swimming pools of London. Knowing of Oliver's love of swimming, Jonathan suggested he ask Oliver about this next time there was an opportunity. The sound man reported back soon afterwards that he had enjoyed a long, fascinating chat with Oliver.

13. When filming in Houston, Oliver came down to breakfast and sat next to Ian. Ian re-members watching Oliver try to open an individual packet of corn flakes. After several minutes of failing, he took a knife to the packet. Ian turned to Oliver and said, "Oliver, you're a cereal killer." Oliver laughed.

14. Beckett S (1938). *Murphy*. Grove Press: New York, p. 37.

15. Merleau-Ponty M (1962). *Phenomenology of Perception*. Routledge: London and The Humanities Press: New York, pp. 137–139, 146, 382–383.

16. Ian's reputation and knowledge about turkeys were going to be recognized at an AGM of the UK Turkey Club when he was due to be elected to the committee. Unfortunately, having driven to the Midlands for the meeting, the building it was held in was not accessible, and Ian could not enter safely. This was not an ideal thing to do to a dis-ability access audit consultant, as they found out. They elected him the next year, (see chapter 8).

17. Bell, C. (1833). *The Hand; its Mechanism and Vital Endowments as Evincing Design*. Bridgewater Treatise, p. 197. Reprinted in 1979 by The Pilgrims Press: Brentwood, UK.

18. Mark Twain once said that the most important people of the nineteenth century were Napoleon and Helen Keller, one for his political life and the other for showing what was possible without two of the six senses, hearing and sight. By those measures Ian, who has studied movement in a way and with an unavoidable intensity and duration matched by few if any others, might be similarly ranked in the twentieth century—with Hitler or Stalin.

19. It was arranged to film Herb Schaumburg after filming with David McNeill in Chicago. Because of the time difference it was necessary to get up at around 4 a.m. to arrive at New York for midday. On arriving at Chicago airport they were waiting when an an-nouncement came over the PA system, "Would Michelle Pfeiffer please go to Gate 13." Every man in the place looked towards the gate. They were met at La Guardia airport by two stretch limos and brought to the front of Herb's hospital. He greeted them warmly and asked if Ian and Jonathan would mind just chatting to a few people before the film-ing began. They trooped into a lecture theater full of doctors, all waiting for them to arrive. Among the audience were Oliver Sacks and the eminent pediatric neurologist, Isobelle Rapin. Ian and Jonathan winged it and then they all had a sandwich. After a

while Herb mentioned casually that he had to leave to pick up his car from the garage in 10 minutes. The crew froze; they had come all that way to film Herb and now he was going. They ran around getting ready at a gallop. Herb turned to Jonathan and said, "That usually gets them moving." In a short interview he was wonderful and much of what he said featured in the *Horizon* film. One bit that did not was when Chris Rawlence asked him, given the severity of Ian's problem and Herb's knowledge of it, how come Ian moved so well. Herb replied, "I have not got a fucking clue."

20. See: http://www.truemovement.net/lessons-from-ian/

Afterwords

1. The Kohnstamm phenomenon involves standing by a wall and typically trying to push one's arm against it hard for 40 seconds or so. Then, afterwards, when the arm is left to relax beside one's chest, it rises up to 45 degrees or so on its own. The aim of the experiments was to see whether peripheral feedback was necessary to the phenomenon. Ian had no rising of the arm.

2. Sacks O (1982). *Awakenings*. Duckworth: London.

3. From Monks R (1990). *Ludwig Wittgenstein: the Duty of Genius*. Jonathan Cape: London. The Feynman quote, "the highest forms of understanding we can achieve are laughter and human compassion," was from Feynman RP (1988). *What Do You Care What Other People Think?* W W Norton: New York.

4. Murphy R (1987). *The Body Silent*. Henry Holt; New York, p. 93.

5. One of these papers is one of Chris's favorite pieces of work (Miall C, Ingram H, Cole J, Gauthier G. The perception of alterations in peripheral weight: a central or peripherally originating task? *Exp Brain Res* 2000;133:491–500). Another paper with him is one of Jonathan's favorites (Miall RC, Cole JD. Evidence for stronger visuo-motor than visuo-proprioceptive conflict during mirror drawing performed by a deafferented subject and control subjects. *Exp Brain Res* 2007;176:432–439).

6. Merleau-Ponty M. (1964). The Primacy of Perception. Northwestern University Press: Chicago, p. 159.

GLOSSARY

Acute sensory neuronopathy syndrome; a rapid onset yet permanent loss of cutaneous touch and proprioception over the body, with loss of reflexes, but without weakness or loss of pain and temperature perception. The cause may be an auto-immune attack on the cell bodies of the nerves underpinning these sensations in the dorsal root ganglia.

Afferent; nerve fibre or axon whose impulses travel from the periphery to the spinal cord and brain. Afferents therefore carry information for sensory perception. In contrast 'efferent' nerves carry impulses away from the brain and are related to movement or motor function.

Allodynia; pain following a stimulus that does not usually provoke pain, here say, after light stroking of the skin.

Ataxia; loss of the coordination and accuracy of movement. When due to sensory loss movements become uncertain and jittery.

Auto-immune disease; a disorder which occurs when the body's immune system attacks and destroys healthy body tissue. Usually the immune system has produced an antibody or immune cells to a foreign cell or infection which then go on to attack specific cells in the body in error.

Axon; the long thin nerve fibres along which nerve impulses are sent. Nerve cells connect with other nerves, or to muscles via specialised junctions called synapses.

Coriolis force; a force on a mass moving in a rotating system which acts perpendicular to the direction of motion. If one sits at the centre of a room rotating clockwise and makes a reaching movement out to the front, then the force from the left will deflect movements to the right.

Cognitive; the acquisition of knowledge and understanding through thought, experience, and the senses, as opposed to that knowledge which appears to be intuitive or beyond our ability to determine its cause, (in education, social skills are sometimes considered non-cognitive).

Cutaneous; relating to the skin.

Cycads; seed plants with a stout, woody trunk and large, hard, stiff, evergreen leaves. They developed at least 280M years ago and have therefore survived essentially unchanged since then, and are found in mainly tropical and subtropical areas.

Deafferentation; loss of afferent nerves. So a large fibre deafferentation leads to a loss of the nerves underpinning the perceptions of touch and proprioception.

Dorsal root ganglion; the small collection of nerve cell bodies (as opposed to the axons of the nerves) just outside the spinal cord in the dorsal or sensory roots of a spinal nerve at each spinal segment. The dorsal root ganglia contain the cell bodies of sensory (afferent) neurons, and if these are damaged then the nerve fibre and its axon no longer works.

Functional imaging; the study of human brain function based on analysis of data acquired using a variety of brain imaging techniques. The most often used is probably functional Magnetic Resonance Imaging (fMRI), but other techniques include Positron Emission Tomography (PET) and Optical Imaging. Electroencephalography (EEG) and Magnetoencephalography (MEG) can also be used. The resolutions in terms of spatial and temporal accuracy of the resulting images differ between techniques.

Gesture; a movement of part of the body, usually the hand or the head, to express an idea or meaning. Here gesture is largely defined as being those movements associated with language. Facial expressions are usually defined as a separate category.

Guillain-Barré Syndrome; a disease with a rapid-onset caused by an auto-immune dysfunction, usually following an infection, leading to damage of the peripheral nervous system. Patients may experience changes in sensation and pain though the main problem is muscle weakness beginning in the feet and hands.

Hyperalgesia; increased pain from a stimulus that usually provokes pain. This is usually after damage or inflammation of the skin. Primary hyperalgesia occurs over the area of damage and occurs to both mechanical and heat stimuli; secondary hyperalgesia is found in a small halo around the injury site and is characterized by mechanical hyperalgesia only.

Insular cortex; (insula, or insular lobe) is an area of cerebral cortex which folds within the lateral sulcus, which separates the temporal lobe from the parietal and frontal lobes. It is thought to have a variety of perceptual and motor roles, including awareness of states of the body such as thirst, hunger, pain, sexual pleasure, bladder fullness and breathlessness which may in turn sum to underpin a sense of body ownership.

On the motor side it may be involved in the cortical control of swallowing, bladder control and stomach motility. It may also be involved in social emotional perception such as some forms of disgust, and empathy.

Laser evoked potentials, LEPs; infrared laser pulses leading to rapid heating of the skin activating heat sensitive skin receptors with a subsequent nerve volley which can be recorded, after a suitable interval, over the opposite cerebral cortex through electrodes placed on the skin of the scalp. Whereas conventional somatosensory evoked potentials (SEP), from low threshold electrical stimulation of the skin, reflect function of large nerve fibers and their pathways to the cortex, temperature and pain perception uses a different set of nerve cells and brain pathways. It is the latter which laser-evoked potentials can investigate and so establish or exclude deficits of Aδ peripheral nerves and of the nociceptive system.

Magneto-encephalography, MEG; a functional neuroimaging technique for mapping brain activity by recording the very small magnetic fields produced by electrical currents occurring naturally in the brain, using highly sensitive magnetometers. The signals are so minute that this has to be done in highly magnetically shielded rooms to exclude extraneous magnetic fields either from electrical sources or from the earth's field.

Morphokinetic; a movement which has accuracy in shape and timing but which does not have to be accurate in place, e.g. a conductor's baton.

Motor cortex; the primary motor cortex, or M1, lies in the frontal lobe of the brain, just anterior to the central gyrus. Its role is to generate neural impulses that control the execution of movement, including its spatiotemporal form and its forces, torques and muscle activity.

Motor program; a neural system for movement control within the brain, so that a given movement is anticipated, planned and guided. Such movements might be called habits or skills, and tend to unfold without voluntary control though thought towards them can be superimposed. Typing and walking, for instance, proceed through motor programs.

Muscle spindle; receptors within muscle that, primarily, respond to change in the length of the muscle and so which can be used by the brain to determine the position and movement of body parts.

Nerve types; Peripheral nerves contain various classes of nerve cell or axon. The largest are the movement or motor nerves starting in the spinal cord and going to muscles. The next largest are the sensory nerves which underpin the sensations of touch and movement/position sense, designated Aβ fibers. The nerve cells in both of these classes are wrapped in a sheath of insulating tissue, myelin, which allows them to conduct fast, at around 50 m/s. Smaller myelinated sensory fibers conducting at 12–20 m/s, Aδ fibers, relay impulses underpinning the perceptions of sharp pain and warmth. The smallest fibers, C fibers, are not myelinated and conduct impulses perceived as duller pain and warmth, at 0.5–2 m/s.

Neuropathy; disease of peripheral nerves. These can involve all fibers, a sensorimotor neuropathy, or preferentially affect motor or sensory nerves. Within sensory neuropathies sometimes larger fibres are affected more, so it presents with loss of touch; if small fibers are affected then awareness of pain and temperature are reduced. Sometimes damaged nerves fire off, so that pins and needles or pain results. Usually a peripheral neuropathy affects the longest and most vulnerable axons first, so symptoms are felt in the feet and hands.

Neuronopathy; Sensory neuronopathies or ganglionopathies result from loss of the nerve cell bodies in the dorsal root ganglia close to the spinal cord at each segmental level, as opposed to loss of the peripheral axons out in the limbs. As a result the sensory loss is usually complete, over body and limbs, rather than being felt more on the distal parts of the arm or leg.

Nociceptive system; the sensory nervous system's response to harmful or potentially harmful stimuli whether chemical (e.g. acid or pepper extract), mechanical (cut, crush or high impact) or thermal (heat and cold). These stimuli excite different classes of high threshold sensory nerve cells called nociceptors which produce signals that travel through specific classes of nerve fibers to the spinal cord and brain. Nociceptive inputs may result in the elaborated subjective experience of pain as well biological and behavioral responses, e.g. reflex withdrawal of a limb.

PET; positive emission tomography; an imaging technique using a radioactive tracer taken up by the brain according to activity within it during a certain test or movement. By recording this and with 3D images of the brain patterns of activation during certain procedures can be measured and compared between and within subjects.

Popperian science; Sir Karl Popper, (1902 – 1994) suggested that a theory in empirical science can never be confirmed, but it can be rejected by falsification. It follows that experiments should be designed to try to falsify a given hypothesis. This is in contrast to less formal experiments guided by informed curiosity which can have unexpected results.

Premotor cortex; an area in the frontal lobe just anterior to the motor cortex itself. The premotor cortex seems to be involved in the selection of, and intention to perform, a particular movement; thus, they seem to be particularly involved in the selection of movements based on external events. The area may be particularly important in translating a verbal or visual cue into a predetermined movement response and in the unfolding of movements from memory.

Proprioception; information arising from joints, muscles and tendons about the movement and position of the body in space and its parts relative to each other. Much of this information is at a level below awareness as the motor system coordinates movement automatically, but we can, of course, attend to movement and position to become aware of some aspects of our proprioceptive information.

Receptive field; the region of sensory space (e.g., on the skin) in which a stimulus will trigger the firing of an individual sensory nerve cell.

Receptor; in the skin, a specialised ending of a sensory nerve which converts a touch, stretch, heat, temperature or nociceptive stimulus into a nerve impulse.

Saccadic eye movements; a fast short movement of both eyes from one fixation point to another. Unlike when an object is tracked by slow pursuit movements of the eyes, the visual images during a saccade are not perceived.

Somatosensory cortex, S1, S2; the sensory cortex lies in the parietal lobe just behind the central sulcus and so abuts the motor cortex anterior to it. The sensory cortex receives sensory information from the body, from its skin, muscles and joints etc. In the first sensory areas, S1, parts of the body are represented in a sequence along the sensory strip, with the foot medially, or near the midline and then the leg, body, arm and face progressively more laterally. The second area, S2, lies behind S1 and may be where the beginning of tactile learning and memory, and discrimination between textures and size of tactile objects occurs, so called higher order processing.

Topokinetic; a movement which has to be accurate in space, especially in relation to an external object or place, e.g. moving to pick up a glass.

Transcranial Magnetic Stimulation, TMS; a magnetic field generator, or "coil", connected to a pulse generator which delivers electric current to the coil, is placed near on the scalp of the subject. When the coil is discharged the magnetic pulse generates a small electric current in the neurons of the brain under the coil via electromagnetic induction. The procedure is generally painless.

Two-alternative forced choice; a method in which during an experiment the subject has to decide between two choices, whether synchronous or asynchronously presented and whether or not she/he perceived those choices consciously.

Vestibular system; structures in the inner ear which underpin the sense of balance and awareness of whole body spatial orientation (right way up or upside-down).

INDEX